Get Off Your Ass!

A book I can recommend without hesitation,
with "both of my thumbs" up!

—WILLIAM LLEWELLYN, OWNER OF MOLECULAR NUTRITION

Tactlessness aside, it's hard to argue with his logic or
the advice [Tuley] offers throughout his book.

—JOHN HANC, *NEW YORK NEWSDAY*

Get Off Your Ass hits you right between the eyes
with a dose of reality . . . and that's much needed in
American society where fraud and deception dominate
the most noble of industries . . . the fitness industry.
Marty speaks to the reader as if he is right there
in the reader's corner, acting as a coach, a trainer,
and an educator. No doubt this book will change lives.

—PHIL KAPLAN, *MIND & MUSCLE FITNESS HOUR RADIO SHOW*

Marty doesn't beat around the bush and he is the
only guy that can tell me to "Get off *my* ass,"
whose ass I won't kick.

—LANA, OWNER OF LANA'S EGG WHITES

Get Off Your Ass!

Marty Tuley is the best kind of iconoclast: He knows
the conventional as well as the unconventional,
and boils it down to the simplest admonition:
"Dude, get it in gear!" He combines logic and passion
in equal doses, and that's an unbeatable combination.

—LOU SCHULER, AUTHOR OF *THE BOOK OF MUSCLE*
AND *THE TESTOSTERONE ADVANTAGE PLAN*

Marty Tuley . . . on one hand . . . a gritty, over the top,
in your face, tell it like it is muscle head akin to a drill sergeant.
On the other . . . a witty, charming, handsome, sincere young
man with a *compelling message,* who truly enjoys nothing
more than being the *catalyst* that changes lives.

—TAMMY PETERSEN, AMERICAN ACADEMY OF HEALTH AND FITNESS

Get Off Your Ass!

The definitive guide to losing weight,
eating healthy, and living longer
. . . for *REAL* people

Marty Tuley

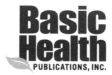
Basic Health
PUBLICATIONS, INC.

The information contained in this book is based upon the research and personal and professional experiences of the author. It is not intended as a substitute for consulting with your physician or other healthcare provider. Any attempt to diagnose and treat an illness should be done under the direction of a healthcare professional.

The publisher does not advocate the use of any particular healthcare protocol but believes the information in this book should be available to the public. The publisher and author are not responsible for any adverse effects or consequences resulting from the use of the suggestions, preparations, or procedures discussed in this book. Should the reader have any questions concerning the appropriateness of any procedures or preparation mentioned, the author and the publisher strongly suggest consulting a professional healthcare advisor.

Basic Health Publications, Inc.
28812 Top of the World Drive
Laguna Beach, CA 92651
949-715-7327

Library of Congress Cataloging-in-Publication Data

Tuley, Marty
    Get off your ass! : the definitive guide to losing weight, eating healthy, and living longer . . . for real people / Marty Tuley.
        p. cm.
    ISBN 1-59120-129-2
    1. Weight loss. 2. Physical fitness. I. Title.

    RM222.2.T796   2005
    613.2'5—dc22
                                                    2004026330

Editor: Chris Mariadason
Copyeditor: Carol Rosenberg
Typesetter: Gary A. Rosenberg
Cover Designer: Mike Stromberg

Printed in the United States of America

10   9   8   7   6   5   4   3   2   1

CONTENTS

This book is dedicated to your past;
remember it, but don't dwell on it.

This book is dedicated to your present;
embrace it with all your passion.

This book is dedicated to your future;
all of its promise, all of its obstacles.

This book is dedicated to YOU!
This is your moment, your life, your chance,
and your opportunity.

Only you can fulfill all its potential:
past, present, and future.

FOREWORD

Johnny Fitness, Editor-in-Chief, *MuscleMag International*

As a man genetically prone to excess body fat (I am the virtual clone of a brother who died prematurely of complications with diabetes brought on by obesity), I welcome any book written by an expert on the power self-motivation can have in weight control. The trouble is that, like an honest politician or an ethical lawyer, self-motivation is hard to find when we need it most. When it comes to finding enough motivation to do the right thing, many of us forever come up short. That's when words, if they're the right words, written with passion by one who knows, can make all the difference.

After a lifetime spent fighting the "Oh, just one more mouthful or two won't hurt" mindset that haunts me whenever mouthwatering food is set before me, I know how difficult it is to push one's chair away from the table. I also know that had I had this book and Marty Tuley's words to guide me years ago, my struggle with overeating and under-exercising would have been different, and a whole lot easier.

Get Off Your Ass is not just another "how to" volume. Not just another "you can if you want to enough" paperback. Author Marty Tuley truly believes, not just in himself, but also in the reader's ability to turn his or her life, health, and weight around for the better. Well written and hard hitting, *Get Off Your Ass* is a must for all who crave change in their lives but don't know how to go about it. I don't doubt that *Get Off Your Ass* will save legions of unhappy overweight people from kicking themselves in the asses after giving way to either overindulgence and/or plain ole laziness. Looked at in that light it could also be a lifesaver . . . and that can't be bad.

How old would you be
if you didn't know how old you are?

—SATCHEL PAIGE (1906–1982)

ACKNOWLEDGMENTS

Thanks, Lovena T. Thanks for "standing by your man."

Thanks, Mom and Dad. You taught me the basics, and gave me the opportunity.

Thanks, Dimitri. Thanks for showing me an unrelenting and unwavering tenacity.

Thanks, Belleville High School. My four years of high school made "me."

Thanks, Steve (Tim). Thanks for getting up with me at 5:00 A.M. to pump iron. I haven't forgotten our deal.

Thanks, C. Moore. Thanks for some sincere, thoughtful, rock-solid advice and friendship when I needed it.

Thanks, Bruce. Thanks for your patience. Thanks for your understanding. Thanks for being my friend.

Thanks, Bob, Dolph, Sandra, Doug, Judy, Bruce . . . thanks to ALL my clients. Thanks for reminding me of the "true" value of fitness.

Thanks, Blitz. Thanks for reminding me daily that life is simple, and simple is all that matters.

Persistence is the twin sister of excellence. One is a matter of quality; the other, a matter of time.

—Marabel Morgan

YOUR CREED

You have made an important decision. You have decided to change your life! You have decided to stop *wishing* you were healthier and instead to do something about it.

Congratulations!

You have decided that you will play ball with your children without getting winded. You have decided to pick out clothes you like, not just ones that fit you. You have decided to ease into a chair, instead of squeeze into it. You have decided to kick, scrape, and fight for every single minute of this life and grab for all the gusto you can because life really is too short.

You have decided that you will not sit around and hope you do not get heart disease, cancer, and/or diabetes. If you sit, you are a target. You have chosen *not* to be a target. You have decided you *will* do everything possible to make sure you don't get caught in the crossfire of disease.

You have decided that you will not do this alone. You will educate your children, your spouse, and your friends about your worthy cause. You will take anyone who will listen and participate along for the ride. You will have a more positive future, because you have decided to . . . **GET OFF YOUR ASS!**

Man who say it cannot be done,
should stay out of the way
of man doing it!

—CHINESE PROVERB

INTRODUCTION

You're Not In Kansas Anymore

STAY ON THE YELLOW BRICK ROAD, meet some good people to help you along your way, and then ask the wizard for directions to Kansas. Isn't that what the good witch told Dorothy to do? You know the story. Oz, Kansas, Dorothy, Toto, Tin Man, Scarecrow, Cowardly Lion. Remember their journey? And ultimately, what did Dorothy discover?

Dorothy learns that essentially what she was looking for was always right there, within her grasp. It turns out Dorothy knew how to get home all along. She just needed a good old-fashioned Midwest twister to teach her what she already knew. Meet your fitness twister.

We (you, me . . . everybody) have entered a completely unknown era of human existence. For the first time since the conception of our species, we must undertake purposeful daily physical activity and regulate our daily nutrition. It really is unparalleled. Think about it. Prior to World War II, almost all jobs in the United States were agricultural and/or physical. Our daily activity and consequent caloric expenditure were things we neither had to consider nor be concerned about. At the same time, our daily diet was limited to our very own production. There were no "quick" shops, monstrous superstores, or fast-food drive-thrus. What we ate was largely what we grew and raised. This meant that indulgences—specifically those associated with eating—were few and far between. Any eating indulgences that did occur were typically part of a holiday celebration or special occasion. Bottom line: we weren't gluttons. But it had more to do with logistics than with self-control.

Inexpensive, low-quality, accessible food is a primary culprit in our obesity epidemic. In the last thirty years alone, the fast-food industry has gone from a $3-billion-a-year industry to a $110-billion-a-year industry! These days food is cheap, convenient, and nutritionally worthless! The fast-food industry's slogan should be TASTES GOOD, KILLS SLOW!

Don't get me wrong. I don't blame the fast-food industry for today's obesity epidemic and neither should you. I believe it would be unfair to do so. The simple fact is we live in a capitalist society, one that is based on supply and demand. I believe the fast-food industry was simply the result of the industrious actions of people who recognized a need in society. Need generates solutions, and solutions come in the form of products sold for profits.

The fact is the fast-food industry has done a good business selling quick, crappy food. What a shocker, right? Wrong. We knew that right out of the gate. So do we really want to admit we are that senseless? Not me, my friend. You knew better and you took it on the chin. Sometimes that happens.

Besides, blaming accomplishes nothing; it certainly won't make you any thinner. Blaming will never be a successful form of exercise. If you choose to blame, you choose to remain fat. Blaming acknowledges your ignorance. You get to be ignorant once, but only once. Ignorance isn't an excuse; it's an acknowledgment, an acknowledgment of your need to learn. I learned.

It took me twelve long years. Twelve years to recognize that health clubs will never solve our obesity epidemic. Twelve years to recognize that selling health club memberships is about making money and living in a nice house and *nothing* about positively changing and improving a person's health and fitness.

Do you think a health club membership will solve your rapidly escalating weight gain? Think again. In 1980, there were approximately 3,000 to 5,000 commercial health clubs in the United States. Today, we have close to 25,000! You'd think we were a country of buff, built bodies. Wrong. During that same time period, obesity rates have almost tripled. So, who's benefiting from all the health clubs?

These days, fast food and health clubs are the least of our problems. We live in a society bent on instant gratification and quick fixes. Seems everybody wants straight white teeth, silky hair, perky boobs, flat stomachs, tight buttocks, nice cars, and big houses. Problem is, no one wants to work for any of these things. Just like our trips to Wal-Mart, we want to "one-stop" shop for everything. We want good, cheap stuff NOW! This is a philosophy and mindset that has carried over to our health and fitness. We've cashed in our dignity and pride for convenience and overnight success. How else would you explain the success of FOX's makeover reality show *The Swan*?

Get Off Your Ass! is your chance for a refund. Your chance to change your attitude, harness your desire, and accomplish something that took some sweat, some really hard work, and a lot of sacrifice. It's your chance to take back your dignity, swallow your pride, and be a role model for your coworkers, your neighbors, your friends, and your family. You can do it. You have it within you. We all do. But it won't happen easily and it won't happen tomorrow. It will be brutally challenging and ego-bruising. It's a voyage that will test your very character.

You'll have to change the very way you view fitness, exercise, and eating right because there is little chance any of us will be returning to the family farm anytime soon. Fitness now becomes synonymous with brushing your teeth. Nobody necessarily likes doing it; we just know we have to.

You can't click your heels to health and fitness. It may have gotten Dorothy home, but it won't get you any thinner. But just like Dorothy, you do have within you the tools for change. In fact, you've always had them. We all do. But we've relegated them to glass boxes with the sign "shatter glass in case of an emergency" while we've hoped and wished for the magic pill, potion, or diet. Well, they're not coming, folks. There's no knight riding a white horse storming toward our castle, and Dorothy has gone back to Kansas. That leaves only me. I am your worst nightmare and your greatest fantasy all at the same time.

Grab your hammer. We've got glass to break!

It's funny about life: if you refuse to accept anything but the very best you will very often get it.

—WILLIAM SOMERSET MAUGHAM

YOU'RE FAT!

YOU'RE FAT! There, I said it. It's out in the open; it's off my chest and yours. Quit avoiding it; just acknowledge the reality. How do I know? Current estimates indicate that 60 percent of Americans are clinically obese. I am surmising that if you picked up this book, you probably fall within that percentage.

"Oh, no, I was just curious."

"Actually, the title caught my attention."

Nice try. No . . . you are probably fat. Okay, *fat* may be too strong a word. I am not trying to offend you, just trying to wake you up! You are not big boned, and it isn't your parents' fault. You're plain old fat. Oops, sorry, there's that word again. It just sounds bad, right? Too personal. Offensive. Great, get a little pissed!

You don't want to be called fat? I don't blame you. Do you want to argue about the offensive nature of the word? Do you want to spend some time discussing the political incorrectness of the term? Sure you do. Do you know why? Because the truth hurts! And it is easier to just sit around and whine about terminology than it is to actually get off your ass and do something about it!

Americans are finger-pointers. If you ask me, it's one of our culture's worst traits. We assume responsibility for as little as possible. It is always someone else's fault. When we spill hot coffee in our laps, we're not clumsy; McDonald's just makes it too hot. It's not our fault our children are becoming more violent; television programming is to blame. Never mind the erosion of the family nucleus.

When we are fat, we label the reasons: it's due to an eating disorder, a self-esteem issue, depression, a thyroid imbalance, slow metabolism, and on and on and on. I don't wish to make light of any of these disorders. These conditions are real and genuine, and some people do indeed suffer from them. But the majority of us do not. The majority of us are lazy, and consequently, fat!

Now the good news: You can do something about it. You can lose 10 pounds; you can lose 100 pounds! But it won't be easy, it won't be quick (nothing worth having ever comes easily or quickly), and you will have to change aspects of your life not for four weeks, twelve weeks, or twenty weeks, but for the rest of your life!

This is **NOT** the "Hollywood Diet"! This is the live-longer and live-better plan. This is the feel-good-about-you program. This is the take-responsibility curriculum. This is . . . *Get Off Your Ass!*

EXCUSES, EXCUSES, EXCUSES!

*"I **don't have** time to exercise."*

*"I **can't afford** a health club membership."*

*"My schedule **won't allow** it."*

*"I work **too late**."*

*"I'm **too tired** when I get home."*

*"The kids keep me **too busy**."*

See, friend, this is where this book and this author are very different from the rest. Richard Simmons I am not. I have written this book hoping that it will inspire, motivate, educate, and support you in your journey to fitness. But ultimately, this is *your* journey! I am not going to hold your hand; no one is. So get over it.

You have to resign YOURSELF to success. You are at a fork in the road. Choose your path, and choose carefully.

Of course you could take the easy path. Stay at home. Continue to gain weight. Continue to be more and more winded from climbing a flight of stairs. Continue to be uncomfortable tying your shoes. Enjoy not having enough energy to play ball with your kid. Forget about ever shopping and buying clothes you actually like. Forget about feeling comfortable in a pair of shorts. Forget about being able to fit into a booth at a restaurant. Look forward to the massive coronary you'll have at fifty-five, which will rob your family and friends of quality years with you. Don't worry about having to drag an oxygen tank with you everywhere you go. Just accept it. Because remember, you chose the path you're on! No, maybe not directly, but certainly indirectly. How? You made choices and decisions concerning your physical activity and your eating habits. The result of those choices is your present physical condition. Do you like what you see? Do you like how you feel?

On the other hand, you could take the more difficult, but ultimately, more rewarding path. This path has benefits that can't be measured, benefits that result in a level of well-being that is "off the charts." The simple fact is that when you feel good, everything is better. EVERYTHING! And why wouldn't it be? Isn't a well-running car that idles quietly, snaps off the line when you hit the accelerator, and has a stereo system that picks up every radio station from here to Mars just a hell of a lot more enjoyable to drive than some broken down jalopy with no heat or air conditioning? Of course it is. That is what fitness can do for you. Turn your jalopy into a ride you can enjoy and consequently make all your journeys and destinations a lot more enjoyable. It's time for a trade-in, my friend. Time to upgrade your Chevy Nova for a fully loaded Lamborghini; spare no expense, after all we're talking about YOU, your body, and your car. Let me help you build a hot rod!

But, hey, I'm going to be right up front with you. This path isn't easy. No bones about it. From a lot of perspectives, the other path is easier and more enjoyable. But be careful, because it's all an illusion. Camouflage. It all feels great until that day: that day when you don't leave the house because you're embarrassed about your size; that night when you no longer go to the movies because you don't fit in the seats; or, God forbid, that moment when you fall to your knees with a massive coronary. All of a sudden, all those years of eating everything you wanted, all those years you skipped exercise for television, suddenly don't seem worth it. Now you find yourself wishing you had all those choices back.

You see, my friend, the second path differs from the first path in two major ways. It gives you:

Greater quantity
and
Better quality
of *life*!

Ultimately, you have only one person in this world to answer to . . . YOURSELF. You have to sleep at night. You have to feel good about yourself. You have to feel good about your decisions. You have to live with your actions. You have to suffer the consequences of your choices. You, you, you, YOU have to decide on the quality of life YOU choose to live! Nobody will decide for you and nobody is to blame for your decisions. Nobody, that is, but YOU!

IT AIN'T ROCKET SCIENCE

Does anyone truly enjoy exercise? Really. I mean, if we didn't have to, would we? Why, because we like to sweat? We like to feel a burn in our lungs, as if we'd swallowed a torch? Because standing in front of a full-length mirror in some ridiculous workout attire repeating a single motion over and over again sounds like a good time?

Hell no! Oh, you've got your maniacs: die-hard runners, bodybuilders, and aerobic queens; those people who spend hours daily toiling at their addiction. But we call them addictions for a reason! How many marathon runners have you seen whose body you'd just die to have? In general, serious runners are excessively thin and have little, if any, significant muscle tone. No one can routinely run as much as it takes to successfully participate in such an event and still maintain a healthy muscle-to-fat ratio.

Don't get me wrong. Does it take an enormous amount of dedication and work to complete a marathon? Of course. Is it an admirable accomplishment? Absolutely. But is it a healthy and viable physical activity for the vast majority of us? Of course not!

Do you think the human body is, in any way, designed or engineered to run twenty-six miles nonstop? No way! Do you have the misconception, as many do, that marathon runners are healthy? They may not be. Running 26 miles, benching 400 pounds, or teaching 15 aerobic classes weekly doesn't necessarily mean you are healthy. Lunatic? Probably. Maniac? Without a doubt. But healthy? Possibly not.

The vast majority of us want three things, and three things only, from exercise. They are not complex and they are not difficult to achieve. They don't involve thousands of dollars in supplements, prescribed meal plans, calorie counting, diet pills, hours spent at some vanity-driven health club, or any worthless exercise equipment marketed through infomercials.

What are these elusive magical health and fitness goals?

- To have more energy

- To feel better

- To look better

It can be done, and I'm going to show you how.

There are three components to a successful health and fitness program. Notice that I didn't say "exercise" program. Why? Because exercise is only one of three components, all of which are necessary to truly change your personal health and fitness level. The other two are nutrition and education. You need all three to really make this wagon role. Each has its value, and each continually contributes to the ultimate success of the others. But, as with anything in life, education is key and *might be* even more important than exercise.

The success of your exercise and the effectiveness of your nutrition are largely based on the quantity and quality of the health and fitness education you acquire. Step one in *any* successful health and fitness plan is education, but a significant amount of the education will take place in the "trenches." Start eating better, start exercising, and start learning!

There are thousands of books on health and fitness out there, and even more opinions. But when it comes right down to it, you could read every book on the shelf and listen to every so-called expert, but it's all worthless if you don't . . . *Get off your ass!*

Everybody wants the degree.
Nobody wants the education.

—DAVE DRAPER, AUTHOR,
BROTHER IRON, SISTER STEEL

THE GOYA HEALTH AND FITNESS PROGRAM

THIS RUN, YOUR RUN, IS COMPOSED OF THREE LAPS. Each lap has its respective role and value. You can't skip a lap. Don't skip a lap. To succeed at this run, you'll need to be diligent and consistent. You can't be diligent, consistent, and skip laps.

Stay the course and remember, in this run, there are no finish lines and no cheering crowds. This is a run that never ends. Once you start running, you will never stop. Your pace may vary, the course may change, but you will not stop. YOU WILL NOT STOP! You are getting off your ass and staying off! Period!

The value of each lap is equal. No one lap is more valuable than another. When you begin to NOT look at the laps individually, but as a whole, you'll begin to understand the strength of the GOYA health and fitness program. You are not doing three laps. You are doing a run. A run comprised of three laps. See the difference? Remember what I said earlier: This is a journey, so quit looking for the finish line.

LAP 1

EDUCATION

IF YOU'RE GONNA DO IT, DO IT RIGHT!

I just can't say it or stress it enough. Successful, long-term weight loss is NOT about the plan, the system, the pill, or a particular piece of fitness equipment. Losing weight and keeping it off is about EDUCATION! EDUCATION!! EDUCATION!!! If you do not continue to educate yourself on aspects of health and fitness, the deck is stacked against you. Why? Because every BODY is different and every BODY will change as they age. Your personal health and fitness needs will change. Your life will change and your health and fitness lifestyle will need to change along with it.

In the natural world, organisms that do not change go extinct. They fail to adapt, and their species is unable to cope with new stimuli, ultimately leading to death. Without continuing education, your health and fitness will go extinct. Think dinosaur—big, bad, and dead! That's not the direction you want to go. You want to be like the small mammal during the decline of the dinosaur, scurrying around on the ground, existing on whatever's available, constantly adapting, constantly learning, and ultimately surviving. That's you. That's me. That's us.

Educate yourself. Continue reading, watching, discussing, and learning about health and fitness, all the while implementing the knowledge you gain. It's the health and fitness soup of life, baby, and your job is to keep stirring, adding, tasting. Do you want to eat one soup the rest of your life? The same soup? Hell no! Educate yourself.

DOING IT WRONG

Where do I start?! By appearances, doing it wrong is damn near the only way exercise and nutrition has ever been done. A single chapter cannot even put a dent in this subject. Doing it wrong should be an epic movie adventure called *Doing It Wrong, Getting Fatter, and Doing It Wrong Again*! How else could you explain our ever-growing belt lines in an equally ever-growing health and fitness industry? Seems to me, if the health and fitness industry were truly providing legitimate solutions to our obesity epidemic, we wouldn't be the fattest country on the planet. Am I right? Of course I am (get used to it).

I'm not going to name names (not too many, at least) but a lot of so-called fitness experts have been endorsing, marketing, and selling a whole lot of snake oil for a whole lot of years. You've been duped about health and fitness for quite some time. But don't blame the industry completely; you've had a hand in the "duping." You've ignored the truth, closed your eyes to the facts, and avoided the application of plain ole common sense for years. You've bought into quick fixes, miraculous cures, and sweat-less exercise. (Sweat-less exercise, are you kidding me?) You've been lazy and you've been unrealistic, and now you've reaped what you've sown. You know where you're at; the question is, where will you go?

I've put together the following sections to provide you with an enjoyable and educational look at some of the most disconcerting issues of the health and fitness industry. Chances are you'll laugh out loud (and I hope you do). But I hope you have a self-deprecating sense of humor, because I can guarantee you'll relate to some of what I'm talking about. You've been there; trust me. Laughing is fine, but please make sure you're also learning. A lot of us have been stepping in the same pile of health and fitness crap for years. Let's start stepping *over* that pile for a change.

WANTED: Role Models!

Studies and polls have indicated that well over 95 percent of the general public knows that regular exercise should be a part of their lives. We can be relatively sure that no one still believes that exercise is a fad or is of no significant long-term benefit. That's a hurdle the fitness industry has jumped. But despite the positive indications of this poll, we can also arrive at an equally disturbing conclusion. If everybody knows they should be exercising, then why is only approximately 10 percent of the population actually practicing regular fitness?

This is a question that needs some serious thought. And to be sure, there is no one easy answer. There are, however, many culprits. And in my opinion, one of the front-runners is our serious lack of exercise professionals who both appear and act in a manner that the general public can relate to and emulate with pride.

I am in no way trying to say that all fitness professionals are unknowledgeable or inexperienced. Nor do I believe that the majority, in any way, act with malice and reckless abandon while promoting or instructing fitness. I'm sure Tony Little (developer and promoter of the Gazelle) is competent, educated, and experienced. Of that I have little (no pun intended) doubt. What I do have a problem with is his approach and his presentation. I'm sure Tony sells a lot of product, but his infomercials rely on cheap thrills and innuendos to make their sales. Also, I find his pushy-used-car salesman persona grating. In my opinion, his approach devalues the fitness industry and the health-and-fitness lifestyle. And just so no one feels left out, Tony Little in no way has the market cornered on this issue.

How about Denise Austin? Without a doubt, she's a sweet person. And I have no qualms about her actual workout instruction. But Denise, if I have to get up one more morning and watch you exercising with a backdrop of white sandy beaches or the Rocky Mountains, I'm going to puke. Get in the world of Middle America, Denise. We work forty to fifty hours a week. We have three kids, a dog, a cat, a mortgage, two car payments, and a view in the morning of a 1970s green shag carpet! Hellooooo!

How about ESPN's *Body Shaping*? A group of middle-aged bodybuilders wearing the latest in spandex "nut-huggers," so tan they look like turnips, with an overcharged "you-can-do-it" aerobic instructor, and two or three fitness models with more plastic than the local recycling center. Is this reality?

Oh, and my personal favorite (unfortunately no longer on the air): *Kiana's Flex Appeal*. The ratings for this show must have been off the charts with the following viewer profile:

Age: sixteen to twenty-five

Sex: male

Daily exercise routine: masturbation!

I loved Kiana's show! But I loved it for the same reasons the above-profiled men did. She trained in a two-piece, Tarzan-want-Jane, fabric-in-short-supply bathing suit! Where do I sign?!

You know who's got a good show? Lee Haney. Ever heard of him? Probably not. Lee's got a little exercise show early in the mornings, during the workweek on some obscure channel with (get this) real people. The backdrops aren't mountains or beaches, and there are no pretty models. There's no bullshit, and no fluff. Lee's message: It takes hard work, consistency, and faith. Now that's groundbreaking.

The critics will have a heyday with my book. For years, I've listened to this orchestra of clowns who still think the Average Joe has a desire to parade around in health clubs wearing makeup and the latest in fitness fashion—or to exercise in their middle-class, picket-fence, two-car garage homes while listening to some silverspooner in front of a tropical backdrop shouting, "You can do it!"

All these so-called "experts" are so tied up in their little worlds that they can't see the forest for the trees. The health and fitness of real people are beginning to mirror their economic and social classes. The "haves" and "have-nots" are becoming the fit and the fat. Ever so slowly, personal health and fitness are becoming the domain of the wealthy and/or famous. Ironically, in a time when our professional athletes are performing at dizzying levels of physical fitness, the spectators are fatter than ever. Shouldn't it be the opposite? Wouldn't you think such marvelous examples of physical fitness would prove inspirational? The general public is not responding and we (the "fitness professionals") have to assume a disproportionate amount of the responsibility.

News bulletin, fitness folks: the majority of you are not helping the fitness cause. You're hindering it!

Gimmicks, Quick Fixes, and Other Crap We See On TV

This topic really doesn't deserve ink! But given how much CRAP relating to fitness, diet, and exercise is sold in this country it must be addressed.

Hint Anything relating to health and fitness sold between midnight and 5 A.M. is crap! Period.

Hint If you are lured to the sale because it's advertised as "no sweat"... *really,* do I have to address this one? Make a note to yourself... you WILL sweat when you exercise! Don't worry about sweating; worry if you're not sweating.

Hint Did you buy a piece of equipment because it "slides easily under your bed"? Once you slid it under, did you ever slide it out again? And if you did, is it now a clothes hanger? Bottom line . . . don't buy equipment for convenience; buy it because it works and you'll work on it!

Hint YOU CANNOT SPOT REDUCE! Repeat. YOU CANNOT SPOT REDUCE! Repeat. YOU CANNOT SPOT REDUCE! Do not spend money on anything that works one muscle or one "problem" part of the body. You could accomplish the same effect and get the same results by writing the check, walking to your toilet, and flushing it to the sea!

Hint Working out at home is NOT convenient. You are NOT more likely to work out because you have equipment in your basement. However, you are more likely to move it from room to room for several years, before either peddling it at a yard sale or throwing it out when you sell the house. (While you might ultimately choose to have exercise equipment in your home and even place it in a convenient space, convenience should be a very small factor in your resolve to exercise or in your decision to purchase equipment.)

Hint If you do buy something from an infomercial, save yourself some time and trouble and immediately place an ad in the paper and see if you can unload your new living room art. If after one week no sucker is found, drag it to the corner on trash day. (We'll call it your first day of exercise.) You'll eventually do it anyway, so get it over with.

Hint No one has ever found fitness or health in a pill. One supplement, one vitamin, one pill won't do it. Good news, the unused nutrients *will* make your urine a vibrant, glow-in-the-dark yellow, which makes late-night bathroom breaks more entertaining. Enjoy.

Hint *Get off your ass!*

Myths of the Midsection

Americans are fixated on the stomach. Why? Well, for most of us this is where a significant portion of our fat is stored. And when a significant amount of it piles up, it doesn't look very good. Plus, when you look at someone, it is completely natural for your eyes, initially, to fall on the midsection. It is the center of our bodies and our eyes are drawn there. Consequently, people spend a lot of time, energy, and money trying to improve this area.

A flat stomach is definitely nice to look at. No question. But, for most of us, it's a "focus" problem, not a stomach problem. Huh? Forget about your stomach. Your stomach isn't the problem. Your stomach is the byproduct of your problem. You want to fix your stomach. But your stomach doesn't need to be fixed. Your head does!

MYTH #1   Crunches will make your stomach flat.

Crunches do not necessarily make your stomach flat. Crunches are an exercise that works the abdominal muscles. Crunches will tone and strengthen your abdominal muscles. But that does not necessarily equate into a flatter, trimmer stomach. However, for a lot of you, it will equate into rug burns and sore necks because you don't do them right.

MYTH #2   500 sit-ups a day will give you a "six-pack."

Traditional sit-ups aren't worthless, but doing 500 a day won't get you that six-pack you want. What it might get you is a sore back and a stiff neck. When performed correctly, sit-ups are just one of the many useful tools in your toolbox. It's not a good idea to put all your energy into one type of exercise, so don't overdo it. (In case you haven't figured this out, 500 is overdoing it.)

MYTH #3   Leg raises are a good lower abdominal exercise.

Leg raises are not an effective lower abdominal exercise, but they are a good hip-flexor exercise. So, if you're looking for some sexy hip-flexors, here's your baby.

MYTH #4 Side crunches are the best exercise for your "love handles."

"Love handles" are fat. You can't exercise fat. If you could, you'd be able to take your fat out for a walk each day.

MYTH #5 Twisting your torso on an exercise machine will work your "love handles."

No. Your body rotates its torso primarily with the muscles of the lower back.

Almost every health club in America has an exercise machine known as the rotary torso. It is one of the most bogus, worthless, and dangerous pieces of exercise equipment ever invented. This is another prime example of the fact that most health clubs are *not* focused on the "true" health and fitness of their members.

MYTH #6 You will get a flat, trim stomach by continuing to search for that one exercise, that one routine, that one product.

You will get that flat, trim stomach only if you . . . *Get off your ass!*

Tanning Salon (a/k/a Cancer Factory)

How did tanning ever become associated with health and fitness? We've heard it before, but just so we are all clear, let's revisit exactly what "tanning" is.

To get a tan is to elicit a response to sunlight (artificial or natural) at the molecular level, causing the outermost layer of skin to darken. This response is the body's natural defense to excessive sunlight (again, artificial or natural).

Defense, you get that? So tanning, for all practical purposes, is a bad thing. Ironic, isn't it, since being tan has become associated with health? Visit any "health" club in America, and more often than not, they offer tanning services to their patrons. Yet another amazing irony since, at their core, health clubs should be providing customers amenities and services that get them healthy, not unhealthy!

In my opinion, tanning is yet another example of how disillusioned our society has become. We'll spend thirty minutes a day tanning our bodies (a medically proven destructive act, exponentially aging our skin), but we won't spend thirty minutes, four days a week, conditioning our bodies and exponentially extending our very lives! You figure it out.

We'll spend more time and money killing ourselves than we will to save our lives. One more time, just to make sure you got that last sentence: *We'll spend more time and money killing ourselves than we will to save ourselves!*

Let's get this straight. We pay to lie in a machine that we know elicits a defensive response from our bodies. But we won't pay to crawl into a machine whose benefits EXTEND our lives? Say what?

I'm not claiming to be a prophet (though the title has a nice ring to it), but mark my words—lawsuits against the tanning industry are coming. It's inevitable. Think about it. You've been lying in a tanning bed for twenty years. You've been tanning two, three, four, and sometimes five times a week. Upon your annual physical, your physician discovers skin cancer, one of the most deadly forms of cancer. Who's to blame? With this country's twisted sense of individual accountability and responsibility, the tanning industry will be to blame. This, despite the fact that, not unlike the tobacco industry, the medical community has said conclusively that tanning is potentially dangerous.

Look, virtually everyone appears (*appears* being the operative word) healthier with a tan. We've been conditioned by Hollywood to believe a bronzed body is attractive and therefore healthier. The truth is, I like how I look with a tan, but as I've mentioned before, this is an issue of priorities. Choosing a tan over exercise is the wrong choice. You can't improve your cardiovascular system by lying in a tanning bed. It may provide you with the illusion of having less fat, but it's just that, an illusion. Quit trying to pull one over on your friends, your coworkers, and most important, yourself.

If you insist on tanning, well then I can't stop you. But just like alcohol consumption, or eating fried foods, or anything where the possibility of an adverse reaction from your choices and actions is evident, think moderation. Think alternative. Think!

Health Clubs . . . What You Need to Know

Health clubs don't work! They never really have and they still don't. I am not saying don't join one; I am saying *know* what you are joining. Believe me, I know! I owned and operated a health club for more than ten years! Here are the facts:

Ninety percent of all new health club members lose interest and quit exercising within ninety days of their membership.

Why? The short answer: health clubs do not get people healthy. If they did, people would stay with it. It's that simple. Instead, health clubs focus on "renting" shiny equipment. The vast majority of health club operators don't care if you know how to use any of it! They are interested in the sale of long-term contracts and then the sale of the next long-term contract.

Health clubs fail (miserably) with one major part of the exercise equation: They do not educate their members!

Without education, members are doomed. Education is the absolute must for successfully maintaining any conditioning program. It's not a unique thought process. It applies to every aspect of our lives. Knowledge is power!

Health clubs are designed and equipped to fill the needs of "fit" people.

What's wrong with that? That group comprises only roughly 3 to 8 percent of the general population. They already know (or at least think they know) what they are doing with regard to exercise. What about the other 92 to 97 percent of us? This is the 90-plus percent that quit exercising within the first ninety days of their health club membership. No support, no education, no success, and no membership.

The cheapest health clubs are the worst health clubs 99 percent of the time!

Why? Because $19.95 a month can't buy you education or support. It isn't economically feasible. You just paid $478.88 ($19.95 x 24 months) for a twelve-cent membership key tag card. Hope it looks good on your key chain.

There are more health clubs than ever before in this country.

Approximately 25,000 by the latest estimates. So if health clubs are doing their jobs, why is obesity at all-time high levels? Why is type 2 diabetes— a condition associated with obesity—at epidemic proportions? WHY IS AMERICA THE FATTEST COUNTRY IN THE WORLD?

70 percent of all new health club members join to lose weight.

So, if seven out of ten people walk through the door to lose weight, why don't health clubs address this issue? Because nutrition is work; it's education; it's expensive. Health clubs attempt to solve your problem with weights and cardio; definitely part of the equation, but hardly all that's needed. Nutrition is at minimum, 50 percent, if not more like 80 percent, of the battle. If you are going to join a health club, join one that specifically addresses nutrition.

Health clubs aren't always to blame.

Do you know why health clubs charge $19.95 a month? It's because you, the consumer, have dictated it. Oh, you're not solely to blame, but you've had a hand in it. How? You made economics the primary consideration in your health club selection. The health-club industry responded with price wars and cheaper and cheaper memberships. It's a "chicken and egg" scenario, but the consumer's decisions, your decisions, have played a role.

Staple What?!

Lately, there has been a strong resurgence in the medical procedure that reduces the size of stomachs. In the last few years, several high-profile celebrities have undergone the knife for purposes of stomach reduction as a "last resort" to weight loss. Let me ask you this: Do alcoholics cut off their hands to avoid drinking?

I am not for stomach reduction. I am not in favor of stapling one of my internal organs. I am not a proponent of placing a rubber band, a piece of string, a plastic tie, or whatever else the medical community may be using to reduce your stomach by strangulation.

"Gosh Doc, lately I just can't seem to get rid of my headaches. Could you cut my head off?"

Sound ridiculous? Of course it does. Why? Because that's not solving a problem; that's eliminating it! Problems not solved, but eliminated, tend to have a way of creeping back into our lives in one form or another.

Here's my real problem with stomach-reducing surgeries. Stomach-reducing surgeries are usually masqueraded as a person's "last option." It's not a person's last option. It is not YOUR last option. There's no such thing. Stomach-reducing surgeries are yet another symptom of a disillusioned society, addicted to instant gratification.

Okay, your weight has gotten out of hand. You're fat, heavy, obese, whatever. It happens. It happened to you. So be it. Your battle, your war, will be waged a little longer than others. It will be a hard-fought engagement indeed. I am envious. Why? Because the spoils of your battle will be that much greater, you don't have farther to go . . . you've got more to gain and a sweeter victory to savor.

Stomach-reducing surgeries are **NOT** your last option!

DOING IT RIGHT!

*Do it right the first time
and you won't have to do it again.*

—PARENTS EVERYWHERE

Sound familiar? Of course it does. This is a line many a mother and father have used again and again with their children. Mine sure did. Our parents were trying to teach us the importance of efficiency and productivity. They knew, as you and I do now, that one wrong step, one skipped step, one short-cut step forward ultimately resulted in the need for two steps back and that often meant you had to start again. The job still had to be done. The only thing you possibly gained was experience and because you tried to "half-ass" it, you probably didn't even get that.

Which means you just completely wasted your most important asset (pun intended)—your time. And that, my friend, is something we get only so much of. It is your most precious commodity, bar none. How you use it, how you spend it, and what you garner from it is all up to you. To add insult to injury, your wrong step, your skipped step, your short cut, and your "half-ass" attempt probably, ultimately, left you with more ass than you started with!

Doing it right is all about attitude, but it has to be the right attitude. An attitude free of excuses and unshackled by past mistakes. An attitude with sails full of wind and sure of direction and driven by the reality that without risk, there is no reward. Look, it's easy to be negative. I've certainly experienced my share. Hell, I have had a bad day or two, even a week, just like the next guy. But I never lost sight of the final objective and during dark times I NEVER shunned the foundational aspects of my life. Figure out what makes up your foundation; build it and maintain it. It will be your bedrock during the storms of your life.

I hope this helps you with your foundation. I hope it makes you think about your attitude and your views. I hope it inspires you, changes you, or simply recharges your batteries. Use this information toward the betterment of your foundation or maybe its maintenance because without your foundation, nothing else matters.

First Things First: Take Some Responsibility!

I've never bought into the argument of the last fifteen years or so about individual lawsuits against the tobacco industry. I have heard all the facts. I understand that the tobacco industry was indeed aware of the addictive nature of its product. Further, it's been conclusively proven that upon their awareness of tobacco's addictive nature, the industry did, indeed, take steps to actually increase the potency of its product.

Okay, that was wrong and the tobacco industry should pay. But in the mid-twentieth century when many social groups began to expound on the dangers of smoking, many of you kept doing it. In the 1970s when the federal government required the tobacco industry to put on the packaging, in no uncertain terms, that smoking was a danger to your health, you kept smoking. You kept smoking right to your deathbed, then you blamed and sued an industry for your choice.

Granted, nicotine is incredibly addictive. Many experts argue it may be one of the most addictive drugs known. But many of you didn't even try to fight. You went right on with a known destructive lifestyle and practice. You went right on indulging in a product you knew was killing you! Killing you! The tobacco industry may be at fault, my friend, but you are also to blame.

I wonder, can someone who dies of liver failure from excessive alcohol consumption sue Budweiser? I hope not.

So who's next? With obesity rapidly closing in on tobacco's number-one position of related deaths a year, where will the finger point next? Look out fast food—here come the lawyers!

No question, the vast majority of food sold (categorized as "fast") is high-calorie, high-sodium, and extensively processed. That's not ground-breaking news, and the fast-food industry has not been covertly in-creasing the calories of meals in an effort to make us a society of obese civilians. Nope, this is plain old capitalism at work. It's called supply and demand. The American consumers have gotten themselves into this mess, and now they will have to get themselves out.

Don't sue the fast-food industry. Don't! You're making the rest of us look like idiots, America . . . the country of finger pointers. It's never our fault, our responsibility, or our problem. Someone else is always to blame.

Take the energy, the time, and the resources you were planning on using in your legal battle with fast food and redirect it. Redirect those resources to changing your life. Get in shape! Form a non-profit organi-zation bent on educating today's youth on better eating habits and the importance of regular exercise. Redirect those resources to make a REAL difference. Do something for yourself or others that brings you pride.

For goodness sake, don't line one more fat-cat attorney's pocket with millions of dollars so that you can get up in front of a jury at the end of a trial and make that oh-so-typical and not so uncommon speech: "I have done this so others like me won't have to suffer."

WHATEVER! Save me your pity, and start exercising!

Big Wars Are Won with Little Battles

The United States has become a society of convenience. Convenience has been aided by ease of transportation and communication. We've shelved neighborhood stores within walking distance for the large one-stop shop. These days it's more convenient and more comfortable to jump in our oversized, gas-guzzling SUVs and drive twenty minutes to a concrete adult playground. I guess the "little guy" didn't carry all the worthless, unnecessary "crap" we thought we needed. So we traded our long-term health and quality of life for big, expensive, environment-destroying SUVs and discount "shit"! Will it be worth it?

SUVs, the environment, and corporate America are issues for another book and another time. The simple fact is, the infrastructure of this country isn't going to change anytime soon. We're a country with large highways, relatively easy means of travel, and (at least for now) inexpensive fuel. Unlike much of Europe and the rest of the world, we are no longer a pedestrian-based society, which means we aren't walking and aren't burning as many calories. To add insult to injury, we coupled our lack of walking with high-calorie, nutritionally low food. We are killing ourselves with convenience, but we don't have to.

We miss a lot of really good exercise opportunities in our everyday lives. We take the elevator instead of the stairs. Granted, if you work on the fortieth floor, no one expects you to take the stairs (unless your name happens to be Lance Armstrong). Here's the Get-Off-Your-Ass rule for stairs: *four floors or less, walk. Five or above, ride. BUT if you do need to go up more than four flights, disembark four floors below your destination and walk the rest.*

We *ride* escalators as opposed to walking on them. Have you ever stopped to watch people riding the escalator? Has it ever dawned on you how silly they look just standing there? No? The next time you're in a department store with an escalator, stop, look, listen. Chances are you'll hear someone complaining that their gym membership dues are too high and they've tried every diet, all the while they're munching on a corn dog and standing on a mechanized system of gears, pulleys, and belts that drags their overweight carcass twenty-some feet off the ground. Don't ride an escalator, walk it!

We drive our car to the gym to exercise, and then bitch if we have to park too far away. Sound familiar? I can't tell you how many times I have heard health club members complain about parking. Or how many times I have watched members circle the lot for that elusive front-row spot, only to walk into the gym and run on a treadmill for thirty minutes!

Do you mow your own lawn? You do? Great. Is it a self-propelled mower? Come on! Push your mower. Break a sweat; maybe even breathe heavily. Pushing your mower won't kill you, but not pushing it may!

Do you drive to places you could probably walk or maybe bike to? Sure you do—we all do. You can't walk or ride all the time, but you *can* do it some of the time. It adds up. It will make a difference, but it starts with choice.

To give you an idea of how it adds up, the following are some common everyday activities ("Get-Off-Your-Ass" activities) and the time it takes to burn 100 calories doing them:

Clean/vacuum/mop floor	25–35 minutes
Wash dishes/iron clothes	45–50 minutes
Mow lawn (self-propelled mower)	25–30 minutes
Mow lawn (manual mower)	12–15 minutes
Gardening (spade/roto-till)	10–20 minutes
Rake leaves	20–25 minutes
Wash/wax car	20–25 minutes
Wash windows	20–30 minutes
Paint (brush)	35–40 minutes
Shovel snow	10–15 minutes
Blow snow	15–20 minutes
Stack firewood	15–20 minutes
Walk (brisk)	15–25 minutes

I know what you are thinking: "Whoopee, 100 calories." Well, yes, but those are 100 calories you're probably not burning now, and it does add up. It is important to understand that most weight gain is cumulative over many years. Though you may think you got fat overnight, I assure you, you did not. It takes years, sometimes decades. It's a snowball effect that starts like this:

You've graduated college and get your first job. You're no longer taking your daily walks to class. This simple, seemingly meaningless lack of activity is resulting in your NOT burning about 200–400 calories a day (that's 1,400–2,800 calories a week). Your new job is rough and demanding, so you've decided to make your career your priority. You "don't have time" for trips to the gym, pick-up basketball, and other physical activities you used to participate in. The loss of those activities is resulting in your not using up another 1,800–3,000 calories a week. To add insult to injury, you're still eating like you're a twenty-year-old college student—skipping breakfast and maybe eating one or two big meals a day. Fast food is still your meal of choice. Oh—and one more thing, you're older now. . . .

Up until you're about twenty-five (give or take a few years) your body keeps up with the aging process by fixing, repairing, and/or replacing more cells than it's losing. However, during your mid-twenties, your body starts losing the battle to Father Time (unless you're exercising regularly and eating right). The result—you're losing muscle and that's a bad, bad thing. Muscle is your engine. It's what keeps your metabolism burning hot. The more muscle, the better (hotter) your metabolism. The less muscle you have, the fewer calories are burned and the more fat you store.

The moral of this story is that you're eating the same way you always have, but you're moving less and getting older. The first year, it's a 3- to 5-pound weight gain. The next year, you lose another 1 percent of your muscle mass, your metabolism slows down a little more, and you gain 5 to 7 more pounds. Ten years after college graduation, your mean, lean 185 pounds is now a jiggly 225. By the time you're in your mid-forties, your weight is 250–260 pounds! Thirty years after college (depending on your genetics and gender), you've gained between 25 and 100 pounds or an average of 3–5 pounds a year. Sound familiar?

Performing simple daily activities can make a difference. As with weight gain, weight loss is also slow and cumulative, so don't run your vacuum and expect to drop 5 pounds. The activities mentioned above burn about 100 calories in the time specified. Review the list and pick out a few you're currently not doing and work them back in your schedule. The result could be another 700–1,400 calories burned a week and the spark of a profound change in your body and your mind. But it starts with a choice . . . choose to *get off your ass*!

Father Time

How old are you? Thirty-five? Forty-five? Fifty-five? Whatever it may be, chances are you're over the "hump." The "hump"? The "hump"—and I am not talking about Wednesday. You've lived more years than you probably have left. Sobering thought, huh?

Has time really gone by that fast? Remember when a year seemed like an eternity? When you lived a lifetime, all in a high-school summer? When college seemed like it would never end? When the "real" world just couldn't and wouldn't come quick enough. And now, it's spinning by so fast you almost feel like you're missing it. The days don't have enough hours and the weeks don't have enough days. You've just celebrated your twenty-, thirty-, or forty-year high-school class reunion. It's all downhill from here. Or is it?

Warriors refuse to grow old gracefully! We're just not going to do it. We're going knuckle-to-knuckle every single step with Father Time. However, when I say put up a fight, I'm not talking toupees and bell-bottoms. I didn't say midlife crisis. Marrying your twenty-year-old assistant doesn't count. I'm not talking about a divorce at forty, a new Harley Davidson, or a membership to the Tan Oasis. Warriors do it tactfully.

Warriors are going to be here to enjoy every single moment with our children. We're going to see them raised happy and healthy. We're going to be there for our grandchildren and our great grandchildren. And that's only the beginning. Father Time will eventually win. But he's going to know he's been in fight!

We're going to treat every obstacle in our lives like a speed bump. We'll slow down, but we're going over. We're going to have regrets because they're inevitable. But we won't dwell on our mistakes or regrets—we just won't repeat them.

One morning you'll wake up and be sixty, seventy, eighty, or ninety years old! "How could it all have happened so fast?" you'll ask. If thirty minutes of exercise three or four days a week (a total of one and a half to two hours) could significantly improve all those years, isn't that a small, small price to pay? Can you even begin to think of any investment with that kind of return?

Put your fists up, Father Time. We're going to the bell!

CHANGING YOUR MINDSET: A TEN-STEP PLAN

You are about to embark on a journey that is, quite frankly, a "hard row to hoe." There will be days, weeks, and even months when you'll want to quit. Make no mistake about it: this is a journey for warriors. There will be few "pats on the back." No "good job" from the sidelines to keep you motivated. No drill sergeant telling you, in no uncertain terms, to get out of bed in the morning. We're no longer in Kansas, Toto.

Many a morning you will be all alone, my friend. Many a day it will just be you and the treadmill at 5:30 in the morning. Yes, this is a lonely, seemingly unappreciated quest. So be it. Warriors don't need cheerleaders.

Hey, I am no Dr. Phil. My college resume includes psychology 101 and I think I got a C. But I do know this, if you're going to change the outside (your body), you have to start with changes to your inside (your mind). I think you can start the process with ten simple, little steps. They seem inconsequential. "Big deal," you'll say. "I *want* to exercise." Well hold on there, pal, you want to drive the car and the wheel hasn't even been invented. As my wife is always quick to point out, even I haven't got them all down. You'll be working on these a while, trust me. Here's the plan:

STEP 1

You no longer sleep in during the workweek. You are up, at the latest, by 6:00 A.M. every morning, earlier if necessary. You go to bed between 10:30 P.M. and midnight, earlier if necessary. You get at least six hours of sleep a night, but absolutely no more than eight. Why? Because warriors know battles are won when you're awake, not asleep. Get up! Life is too short. You'll never die wishing you'd slept more!

STEP 2

You read every night for thirty minutes. Not *Cosmo* and not *Sports Illustrated*. Pick something that will make you a better employee, a better spouse, a better father, a better mother, a BETTER PERSON.

STEP 3

Either Saturday or Sunday, you can sleep in until 9:00 or 10:00 A.M. It's okay to stay up late occasionally, have a few drinks, and eat something deep fried. No problem. You're eating better, exercising regularly, but you're no maniac. Life is still for living, and it's all about balance and moderation.

STEP 4

When your alarm goes off in the morning, do the following: Sit up on the side of your bed. Stretch. Yawn. Pet your dog. Kiss your spouse. Smile! MILLIONS of people would give anything to be in your shoes.

STEP 5

You arrive at work every day at least fifteen minutes early. Why? Because if you're going to do something for eight to ten hours, you're going to do it right, do it with pride, and do it to the best of your ability. Slackers walk into work at five after nine. Your job may be to pour coffee at a convenience store, but you will be the best damn coffee pourer west of the Mississippi. Warriors wouldn't do it any other way.

STEP 6

You will work at least forty hours a week, but no more than fifty hours a week. If your career or boss demands more than fifty hours a week, one of the following is occurring:

You're not utilizing your time effectively or efficiently.

You're probably on your second, third, or fourth spouse.

You may have children and family, but you don't know most of them by name.

You're a miserable SOB with no real, genuine friends or social life.

You need a new career (but until that new career comes along, you'll do the one you have at a 110 percent).

and

You're probably fat and out of shape.

Are you getting paid enough for this fine life you've carved up?

STEP 7

When you leave work, you LEAVE work. No cell phones and no pagers; you're not that important. Get over yourself, and give us all a break.

STEP 8

You WILL NOT piss and moan about anything! It does no good. Instead, do something about it! Think life dealt you a bad hand? Don't just demand a re-deal . . . warriors demand a new deck of cards!

STEP 9

Practice empathy. It's probably the most elusive, least-practiced, and most-ignored exercise in humanity. No, not sympathy. Try to really understand the other person. Put yourself in their shoes. It's not enough to sympathize. Ask yourself, "Why is he or she that way?" "What makes my neighbor take the position he or she does?" "What has happened to make my coworker feel or act in that manner?" When you can effectively empathize with your coworker, your neighbor, your spouse, and your children, you've reached a new level of understanding.

STEP 10

Follow all of the above for one full month before you start *anything* else, including exercise, and then *get off your ass!*

NIKE SAID IT BEST

I expect a lot of criticism for some of my suggestions and positions on various facets of fitness discussed in this book. The first idea to be torn apart will most likely be that the exercise portion of the GOYA program initially involves only thirty minutes of exercise twice a week for the first four weeks! The fitness people will shout, "How could that be of any benefit?! No one will ever see results with one workout a week!"

It's a radical suggestion, I'll admit, differing greatly from conventional wisdom and "expert" advice. And, in terms of initially accomplishing measurable physical results, Lap Two alone won't get it done.

My wife (a die-hard fitness enthusiast) argued that people won't stick with an exercise plan if they don't see results. That does seem logical. But look at the reality: Result-driven exercise routines, equipment, and diets are all we've had for twenty years and where has it gotten us? Obesity levels are off the charts and at all-time highs. Heart disease, diabetes, and literally hundreds of other obesity-related disorders are on the rise. So results and success have, in fact, not provided the necessary motivation for long-term health and fitness success.

I wrote this book and its exercise plan from the perspective of the "Average Joe and Jane," that guy or gal out there who is thirty-plus years old, 20–150 (or more) pounds overweight, and has never really consciously exercised. I want them to read this book and say, "I can do that! I can start with one day a week." I want them to, first and foremost, develop the habits. I don't want them looking for results. Results will come, but first learn to just drag your ass out of bed. In other words, think *habit*, not *results*. For a lot of us, this is the real battle. We can all exercise; we just have to get there. It's like learning to take a left at Subway instead of a right at McDonald's.

The richest people in the world didn't get rich quick. It didn't happen overnight, and it didn't happen by purchasing some late-night, get-rich "kit." It came by toiling for hours, days, weeks, years, decades, and even lifetimes. It came, often without success, and, many times, it was preceded by failure. Most people are looking for the finish line. Start paying attention to the journey. Physical, measurable fitness success won't get it done. Seeing results isn't enough. Drop your dependency on the idea that results are necessary in order to succeed. The two are not necessarily intertwined. You simply have to resign yourself to the reality that exercise has to be, must be, a part of your life. You have no choice. Don't debate it. Don't argue it. Nike did say it best: "Just do it!" But in order to "Just do it," you have to first get off your ass!

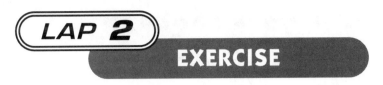

Hundreds and thousands of pages have been written on the subject of exercise. With me, you get one short chapter. Too much has been written on this subject anyway, way too much. Everybody wants to make it too complex. Everybody is searching for the one machine, the one routine, the one philosophy. If you're a searcher, you're a slacker. Quit being a searcher and quit being a slacker! Deep down in your gut, you know if it sounds too good to be true, it is. So quit searching, quit slacking, and pour yourself a BIG cup of Get Off Your Ass! Let's talk about the "ideal" candidates for the GOYA program.

Age 24–64: Any younger or older, and you know it all.

Exercise history: Little or none. (If you have some, all I ask is that you clear your mind and learn.)

Gender: Doesn't matter. (Quite frankly, men, women are better listeners. Take a lesson from our better half.)

Weight: Over. Enough said.

Determination: Off the scale!

Fortitude: Too high to measure!

Resolve: If you were an element, you'd be IRON!

In short, if you've got a pulse and an attitude, you're in!

There are really just two components of an exercise program: resistance training and cardio conditioning. There are a lot of ways to "skin the cat," but here's how I skin the old feline.

Baby steps! Most people decide to change their lives, and start off with five days a week of exercise and some sort of torturous diet! Initially, everyone hangs on for a while. But ultimately, virtually everyone fails. Why? You've set yourself up for it. You've crammed too much on your plate and made it impossible to achieve any lasting, long-term success.

GOYA is different.

THE GOYA PROGRAM

THE FIRST MONTH

For the first month, I'm only asking you to get up and exercise *eight* times. Yes, only eight times in one month, giving you a total exercise time of approximately three hours! Tell me you don't have time for that, and I will personally visit you and pin an official "Lazy Ass" button on your chest.

Trust me . . . work out first thing in the morning. Get it done, get it out of the way, and get the day started with a skip, not a foot-dragging lurch.

I suggest that you work out between 5:00 A.M. and 7:30 A.M.—maybe even 8:30 A.M. It really depends on your daily schedule. The point is—at least initially—exercise first thing in the morning. True, I don't work out in the morning, but I've already developed a regular exercise habit and I never let myself down. You're not there yet; you're just starting to develop the habit of exercise. So, you'll need to avoid any potential obstacles—one of the biggest being procrastination. The further into your day you get without exercising, the less likely you will get around to it. All day long you'll be telling yourself that you'll exercise later, but later never comes. It evolves into tomorrow and tomorrow becomes the next day and the next day becomes next week. Before you know it, you've quit what you never started. It won't be easy getting up a little earlier than you normally would to exercise, but the truth is, you'll feel a hell of a lot better mentally, emotionally, and physically if you exercise first thing in the morning. Get up and start the habit. Forget the snooze button. Just GET UP! Forget the snooze button! GET UP!

So, you know what time you'll be exercising (between 5:00 A.M. and 8:30 A.M.). The days you'll be exercising are Monday and Thursday. Why Monday and Thursday? Well, there are several reasons, some of them psychological and some of them physical.

Start your week on a positive note, hence Monday. It's the beginning; get up, get a sweat going, and begin the day with a positive experience. Start the day doing something rewarding. You'll spend much of your week doing something for somebody else, so give yourself a little something first. Working out on Monday will put a little spring in your step.

Your second workout is Thursday. You could do it on Friday; either day works from the perspective of physical rest because, initially, you'll need two to three days rest between workouts. However, Fridays are often mentally rolled into weekends and your mind may already be a day ahead of your body. Additionally, Fridays are often travel days for three-day weekends, and this sometimes means you'll use it as justification for skipping your exercise. So, for the most part, work out on Thursday and don't give yourself the "travel loophole" or any other excuse. Here's your routine:

Cardio

There are a lot of ways to get your cardio conditioning; run, walk, stairs, bicycling, and so on. But let's face it, and let's be honest. Though convenience shouldn't be your only factor with regard to exercise selection, it should be a consideration. That doesn't mean grab your Visa, turn on the Home Shopping Channel, and buy that piece of equipment that folds ten different ways sideways and conveniently fits into a shoebox. It means that before you use your body, use your brain. Do your research, and consider purchasing a legitimate piece of exercise equipment from a reputable company. Having the proper piece of cardiovascular equipment conveniently located bedside can make a difference. I do my cardio on the Precor Elliptical Fitness Crosstrainer (visit www.precor.com).

Precor is a long-standing company whose history includes the distinction of being the innovator of the elliptical concept. The elliptical motion is a vastly superior form of cardiovascular exercise, which eliminates body-weight impact on the joints and greatly increases the range of motion of the knees and hips. More range of motion means more muscle utilized, which translates into more calories burned.

I'm not particular on the type of cardio you choose to do, so it's not imperative that you go out and buy a piece of cardio equipment. In fact, I'd actually prefer that you spread the love around and do several different types of cardio. Here are some ideas:

Walk your dog. Your dog also needs regular exercise, so use him or her to help yourself, and "kill two birds with one stone."

Power walk. Power walking is an excellent form of cardio conditioning. Swing your arms forcefully and walk as fast as you comfortably can. (You could also do this while walking your dog.)

Walk, sprint, or run stairs. I am a huge fan of stairs. Because you're body is on an incline as you exercise, you're placing a considerable amount of resistance on your legs, not to mention a pronounced range of motion. And you do it all with little or no destructive impact to your knees, lower back, or hips.

Bike. Here's another goodie. Biking (inside or out) has all the benefits of using stairs. Assuming you're not on a stationary bike, it also has the potential for improved scenery.

Don't Run!

When I say "run" here, I'm talking about that ridiculous form of ancient, ignorant self-torture still practiced by way too many people in this modern day and age. Can you tell I'm not a fan of running?

Do you know why running is so popular? Because it's fun, right? Are you kidding me? Because it's easy? Hell no, in fact, it's hard, too hard (more on that later). Running is popular because anybody can do it. All you really need are two working legs. You don't need a gym membership, expert training, and/or equipment in your basement. Running is a popular form of exercise by simple default. People run because they can, and herein lies my problem. That's just not a good enough reason.

Look, I take my hat off to anyone who exercises regularly, even if their preferred form of exercise is running. I applaud any and all of those people who are courageous enough to take on some form of exercise to improve their lives. A friend of mine recently shed about 30 pounds by running regularly. He was inspired by the Get-Off-Your-Ass message, and that's exactly what he did. He's now preparing for the Chicago Marathon! Admirable, to say the least. Regular exercise is a tough step, and if you've successfully taken it (as my friend did), for God's sake, don't stop. Don't stop, but do think about what you're doing. Now that you're up and at it (whatever "it" is), why not make sure what you're doing is really providing you the maximum benefit with the minimum expense.

Running is terribly destructive to the body. It beats your hip, knee,

Jump rope. Here's a long-forgotten, fallen-out-of-vogue form of cardio conditioning that is inexpensive, simple, and effective. Jump rope any way you can. You don't have to look like Rocky while you're doing it; just get your carcass over the rope.

Walk on a treadmill. Walk, don't run, and be sure to use the incline. Walking at an incline on a treadmill may be boring, but it is effective.

Combine a couple of the above for a varied workout—for example, ten

and lower back joints to a pulp. Run consistently for twenty or so years and tell me how those joints feel. Long-term, consistent running also leads to poor posture. Running exacerbates the rounding forward of the shoulders. This leads to the elongation of the upper back muscles and the shortening of the upper chest muscles. For people who have been running for years, decades, or life, this type of posture is very difficult to correct. Bad posture isn't just cosmetic. It exacerbates a host of other physical problems; including lower back pain, breathing difficulties, and circulation problems, to name a few.

Okay, okay, let me cut to the chase. If you enjoy running and I can't talk you out of it, run only occasionally as part of your health and fitness lifestyle, especially when the weather is mild. Also, instead of mindlessly pounding the pavement for miles and hours on end, consider using a little gray matter, and try running stairs and/or sprinting.

Running stairs requires a much greater range of motion of the hips and knees, without the destructive pounding of your body weight. The increased range of motion means that you're utilizing more muscles and recruiting the usage of more muscle motor units. That's a good thing. This is because the more muscles that are involved, the more calories you'll burn. And for the vast majority of us, that's what exercise is all about. The rule with stairs is to run up and walk down.

Consider performing your running in a sprint/rest format. Think in terms of sets, not time or miles. Twenty-, forty-, and sixty-yard sprints back to back with limited rest periods are an excellent form of cardio conditioning.

minutes of walking and ten minutes of jumping rope, whatever—the bottom line is . . . just make sure you do ten minutes of cardio consistently.

The two goals for your first month of cardio exercise are 1) Do it! and 2) Give me ten total minutes at a moderate work level twice a week. "How do I know if I'm exercising at a *moderate* work level?" you ask. First, forget about monitoring your pulse. I know, I know. That flies in the eyes of conventional wisdom. For years you've been hearing about the "optimum fat-burning zone," your "target heart rate," and so on. These can be effective tools, but I won't get into the specifics of their calculations or their use. Why? Because I wrote the GOYA program specifically for you—a person who has never exercised or hasn't done so in a very long time—and I want you to learn what I believe is the most important aspect of successful health and fitness. Learn to listen to your body. You don't need a heart-rate chart or a heart monitor; you've already got both, your BRAIN! Use it.

So when your brain recognizes that you're breathing at a quicker rate than if you were sitting in your lounge chair (but you're not coughing up a lung), and you have maybe a few drops of sweat on your brow, you're probably exercising at a moderate level. Don't make it any more complex than that.

Resistance

Four body-weight exercises and ten more minutes of your time. Do each of the following exercises for **two sets** of twelve repetitions and rest twenty to thirty seconds between sets. (See Appendix B for photos and detailed descriptions of exercises.)

Sumo Chair Squats

Superman

Pyramid Push-ups

Head and Shoulder Curl

First Month—Quick Recap

Two workouts a week for the first four weeks.

Work out between 5:00 A.M. and 8:30 A.M. on Monday and Thursday.

First do your cardio conditioning.

Do ten minutes of moderate cardio and no more. Could you do more? Probably. But that's not the point. The point is habit and consistency. Stay the course!

Four body-weight exercises for two sets of twelve repetitions with twenty seconds rest between sets.

THE SECOND MONTH

Now we begin "ratcheting" things up a bit. BUT just a bit mind you. You're in a hurry, I know. But Rome wasn't built in a day and neither are you. As I've said all along, quit thinking *destination* and start thinking *journey*!

The basics stay the same with just some *little* twists. Here's your "twist list" for the next four weeks:

1. Increase your cardio exercise time from ten minutes to fifteen minutes, but still at only a moderate work level.

2. Add the following body-weight exercise to the other four you've already been doing and increase your repetitions on all of the exercises from twelve to fifteen.

   Arm circles

3. Add another day of exercise to your weekly routine. That's right. Another WHOLE thirty minutes of exercise a week! Where will you find the time? Funny you should ask. You'll find that extra time between 5:00 A.M. and 8:30 A.M. on Wednesday mornings. Now that you're adding a new day of exercise and have gotten into the habit of working out, you will also move your Thursday exercise day to Friday.

Second Month—Quick Recap

Increase your cardio from ten minutes to fifteen total minutes, keeping your intensity at a moderate level.

Add another body-weight exercise and increase the repetitions on all the exercises from twelve to fifteen.

- Sumo Chair Squats

- Superman

- Pyramid Push-ups

- Head and Shoulder Curl

- Arm Circles (new)

- Add another day of exercise. You now work out Monday, Wednesday, and Friday (instead of Thursday) mornings. In the event weekend plans make it unlikely you'll work out on Friday morning, do your Friday workout on Thursday morning. DON'T MISS WORKOUTS. EVER!

THE THIRD MONTH

Okay, you're getting ready to start month three. Congratulations! You're on the path, you're taking the journey, and you're changing your life! That's not just some little old thing. That's some sh!t! Changing *any* element of your life is tough stuff. Stand a little taller. Lift your chest a little higher. You're in the battle—now keep swinging that sword.

In month three, I need you to spend a little money. Not much, but a little. Trust me, you'll be spending money on the tried and true. Not some fly-by-night piece-of-crap exercise equipment that won't even make it to the next trash day.

Nope, I'm asking you to purchase the "old faithful" of exercise equipment. Nothing fancy, no bells or whistles, it doesn't vibrate, won't slip easily under the bed, and you can't buy it late at night with some supermodel's stamp of approval. BUT it is time tested and has more research behind it than any other piece of exercise equipment currently available and will last you a lifetime. Better value you simply cannot find.

I need you to buy an adjustable set of dumbbells and a multipurpose flat bench. These are not unique pieces of equipment. You can get them at almost any sporting-good store or even large discount stores. Where do I recommend you make your purchase? The York Barbell Company. Why? Simple. The York Barbell Company (www.yorkbarbell.com) has been around since 1932! That's consistency. Its founder, Bob Hoffman, is a virtual legend in the fitness world and is aptly referred to as "the father of weightlifting."

You'll be utilizing your new weight equipment twice a week, Monday and Friday. On Wednesday, you'll still be doing your fifteen minutes of moderate-intensity cardio and your five body-weight exercises now for three sets of fifteen (up until this point, you've only been doing two total sets).

However, on Monday and Friday "things" are changing. You'll still need to do your fifteen minutes of moderate-intensity cardio. This is the same old, same old. You'll want to do more cardio, but refrain. You can add more later, but at this point, fifteen minutes is all the "doctor" is asking for. Remember . . . baby steps, baby steps. It's about starting the habit of exercise.

Here's your resistance routine. (Detailed descriptions of these exercises can be found in Appendix B.)

Flat Bench Dumbbell Presses

Standing Overhead Dumbbell Presses

Two Arm Dumbbell Rows

Bench Squats

Butt-ups with Reach-Through Crunches

You'll do two sets of twelve to fifteen repetitions with twenty to thirty seconds rest between sets. Don't kill yourself with the amount of weight you lift, but at the same time, it shouldn't be a walk in the park either. Choose a weight that will allow you to achieve ten to twelve repetitions with proper form.

It's all about form. Forget everything else you think you know about exercise, because it all starts with proper form and exercise execution. It's the "means" that justify the "ends," and in this case, in your case, the means is the form you use in exercise.

I put very little emphasis or explanation on the amount of weight you should lift. There's a reason for this: the amount of weight you ultimately or initially lift depends on your form. Any weight-lifting increases you experience as you exercise and move along in your journey to fitness are the byproduct of proper form. In other words, forget about how much weight you're lifting, could lift, or will lift. It's irrelevant. First, before any-thing else, you *must* do the exercises correctly. If you do, and you're con-sistent, you will get stronger, but only as a direct result of your form, not vice versa.

The Third Month—Quick Recap

Do your fifteen minutes of cardio every exercise day.

Replace the body-weight exercises on Mondays and Fridays with weight-training exercises. Wednesdays stay the same.

Carefully review all the descriptions and photographs in Appendix B to ensure you have a grasp and understanding of the motions. Per-form the exercises exactly as shown.

Control the movement. The positive (up) and negative (down) aspects

How Much Weight Should I Lift?

I can't tell you how much weight to lift without actually meeting and working with you. You'll need to determine how much weight to lift without the benefit of my simply telling you. But don't sweat it; it's really pretty simple to figure out for yourself.

Each repetition has a positive (concentric) and negative (eccen-tric) aspect. The positive aspect involves a muscle contraction; the negative involves resisting and stretching. Pushing a weight up is the positive aspect; coming down is the negative aspect. Both are *equally* important.

On every resistance exercise you do in the GOYA program, I want you to perform a slow count of 1–2–3 up and a slow count of 1–2–3 down. You'll be doing this for fifteen total repetitions. How much weight you use depends on the maintenance of this count during the exercises. If you can't do fifteen total repetitions and maintain the count, you're training with weights that are too heavy for you. If you do fifteen repetitions, but know you could have done twenty, you need heavier weights. Isn't that simple? See why form dictates the amount of weight you use and not vice versa?

of the exercises should be at the same speed, SLOW! A slow count of three on the way down and up.

Forget about the amount of weight you're using. First and foremost, learn to "feel" your muscles to determine the proper weight.

For all exercises, do two sets of twelve to fifteen repetitions.

Rest only twenty to thirty seconds between sets.

THE FOURTH MONTH

Well, here we are. This is what I like to call the "90 day hump." Studies show that more than 90 percent of the people who undertake a new nutritional plan (diet), exercise routine, or both fail within the first ninety days. Are you one of them? Will you be one of them?

NO! HELL NO! You will not. You have resigned yourself to the habit of exercise. You've decided to make a positive change in your life! Not for a month, not for a year, but forever! You've decided to be a model for your children, your spouse, your family, your friends, your UPS man, and so on.

You're not looking for the quick fix or short-term results. You're not chasing the rainbow for the pot of gold. You're enjoying the rainbow.

There's only one change in routine this month; just add one more set to your resistance exercises for a total of three sets. Everything else stays the same.

The Fourth Month—Quick Recap

Do your fifteen minutes of cardio first.

Doing your cardio is important, BUT it is not more important than weight resistance. DO NOT sacrifice your weights for more cardio time.

Perform the exercises exactly as shown in Appendix B.

For all exercises, do *three* sets of twelve to fifteen repetitions.

Rest only twenty to thirty seconds between sets.

Perform your body-weight exercises on Wednesday.

Don't miss workouts ever. If you need to take a morning off, make it up the following morning. In other words, do the workout you missed the very next day.

You can probably come up with an excuse not to do a particular workout every single day of your life. 99.9 percent of those excuses are complete CRAP, and you know it. Don't fall prey to excuses!

GOYA PROGRAM SUMMARY

The First Month

Exercise first thing in the morning between 5:00 A.M. and 8:30 A.M.

Work out on Monday and Thursday mornings.

Do ten minutes of cardio at a moderate work level.

Do four body-weight exercises for two sets of twelve repetitions with twenty to thirty seconds rest between.

The Second Month

Increase your moderate-intensity cardio from ten minutes to fifteen minutes.

Add one additional body-weight exercise.

Increase your repetitions from twelve to fifteen on all your body-weight exercises.

Add another morning of exercise. Switch your workout days from Monday and Thursday to Monday, Wednesday, and Friday.

The Third Month

Continue doing fifteen minutes of moderate-intensity cardio.

Switch from body-weight exercises on Monday and Friday to the six basic weight-training exercises for two sets of twelve each.

Continue doing your body-weight exercises for three sets of fifteen on Wednesday.

The Fourth Month

- Continue doing your moderate-intensity cardio for fifteen minutes.
- Continue doing your body-weight exercise on Wednesday for three sets of fifteen each.
- Add one additional set to your weight-resistance exercises, on Monday and Friday, for a total of three sets.

I can't say this enough: *Think habit, NOT results.* Results are inevitable if you maintain a consistent exercise routine. Trust me . . . if you get off your ass regularly, changes *will* happen. So quit being fixated on them! They're coming. Instead, learn to appreciate, enjoy, and *respect* the journey of fitness for what it is. Following the GOYA program is an effort in dedication and discipline for those who are strong in heart and mind, and willingly ready to accept the challenge offered and the rewards reaped. You *can* do it!

IT'S WEIGHT-*FEELING!* NOT WEIGHT-*LIFTING*

Things got screwed up right from the beginning. No one stopped to think or consider the ramifications of using the term *weightlifting*. No, no, no, we just jumped right in, put two words together, and gave it absolutely no serious mental strain. Big mistake!

I hate the term *weightlifting*. It has made my job—the job of a health and fitness educator—considerably harder. A lot harder! Now, granted, the term *weightlifting* by itself is not actually (by definition) incorrect. You could argue pretty successfully that is does indeed describe the action, but therein lies the problem. Most of us don't perform the activity of weightlifting correctly. If we did, if we had from the beginning, it would be called weight-*feeling*.

So, why is the term *weightlifting* incorrect? Because the term is generic; we lift weights all day long. We lift bags of groceries. We lift luggage. We lift our pets or children. We lift our garbage. We lift our garage doors. We lift our asses. And so on. In all of the above cases, we are lifting weight. We are moving an object from point A to point B. In all of these examples, we're weightlifting.

Do you see why the term *weightlifting* is all wrong for exercise? We simply applied the same basic logic to the action of exercise that we did to moving the "crap" around in our daily lives. We decided that moving a weight from point A to point B was all that exercising with weights was about. We decided that lifting our garbage and lifting a dumbbell were one in the same. We decided that they were largely the same activity and largely of the same value. Wrong!

Pay attention! Pay attention to your body when you're exercising with weights. Learn to listen to your body. Trust me, it's talking; you just can't hear it. You're not listening. The body is wired top to bottom. Your nervous system is the most intricate, sophisticated network of communication ever built. It makes the Internet look like an eighth-grade science project. But, like anything, lack of use results in a lack of production. Start using your communication system.

When you exercise with weights, your brain sends out a "contract" signal to all relevant muscles. That signal is sent via the nerve cells that make up the nervous system. The relaying of that signal down your nervous system is exercise for your nerves; in the beginning, your nerve cells are not that good at delivering a clear and precise message. Your nerve cells are out of shape. This is one of the reasons why exercising is harder for beginners.

It sounds silly, but visualize the muscles you're using when you're exercising. Simply try to picture the muscle working. Keep the motion slow, distinct, direct, and controlled. This will help you learn to *feel* and become accustomed to the action of your muscles.

Over time, your nerve cells will become increasingly adept at delivering a strong and complete message to your muscles. Over time, you'll learn to *feel* the weight being lifted. Then, you'll be well on your way to becoming a good weight-*feeler*!

CONSISTENCY IS KEY!

Think working out is hard? Wrong! Sticking with it is. Consistency is the key to both achieving and maintaining long-term positive health and fitness changes. Regular exercise is a pain in the ass! But it's a necessity. I hope by now I'm beginning to convince you of that. Because the bottom line is: you don't have to *like* working out, you've just got to do it!

Think about how many things in life we don't like, but we do anyway. We don't like to pay taxes. We pay taxes so that we have modern highways, good schools, government programs, national defense, social security, and so on. A lot of us don't even like going to work. Many of us work to *live*. We put in our eight hours a day purely to ensure that we can enjoy the hours we don't work. We don't like to mow the lawn, but we like the way a well-manicured lawn looks. We don't like to take out the trash, but we like the way our trash-free kitchens smell.

We spend a lot of time doing things we don't like. But by their completion, we ensure ourselves the ability, the time, and the resources to do the things we do enjoy.

Diligence is the mother of good luck.

—BENJAMIN FRANKLIN

Regular exercise is one of those things. You will eventually learn to enjoy exercise, but you may never like having to do it. And there will be many a day, many a morning, when you won't want to do it. Those mornings will come tomorrow, five years, and even twenty years from now.

Trust me, I know. As I sit hear writing these words, I'm thinking about my pending workout. It's Sunday, it's snowing, it's cold, I'm tired, and do you think for a New-York minute I want to exercise? Hell no! But I will; it's a habit I've cultivated over the years.

Indeed, some of those days you may just skip your workout. That's okay. Because the vast majority of the time you'll get up, pour that cup of coffee, and hit the treadmill. The vast majority of the time, you'll grab the leash, the family pooch, and beat the sidewalk. The vast majority of the time, you'll dress, get in the car, drive across town, and walk the old high-school stadium stairs. The vast majority of the time you'll use that health club membership. Because, the vast majority of the time, you'll **get off your ass!**

Habit and Health

by Dr. Frank Crane

The following article appeared in a late 1930s health and fitness magazine. How quick we are to forget what we would already know. Let's stop making mistakes with regard to our health and fitness by simply not repeating old ones.

The foundation of health is habit.

No new system, whether of medicine or exercise, will do you permanent good. At least, not until it has been followed long enough to become an old system.

For every man that has lost his life by what he did in the last five minutes, a hundred men have died because of what they have been doing the last five years.

Nature has usually enough resiliency to resist any sudden assault, and we recover from a fall of a fever, but it is the slow gnawing of long bad habits that honeycombs our strength and brings on our ruin.

So if you are taking up any scheme of exercise for your health, do not look for any returns until the thirtieth day.

Also, no exercise is of real value so long as it is conscious. Consciousness of effort is a sign of imperfection. Notice a musician who is a master. He seems to make no effort. In fact we call a perfect piano performance "playing" the piano. When you say the pianist "works" at it, you slur him.

When you try to think and work in ill health, what a struggle it is! You are conscious of tense effort to keep yourself up to the mark. But when you are well and strong all is easy. To be lasting value, then, any exercise must be kept up regularly until it passes from the conscious down into the subconscious, and we can do it, not thinking of it.

And it must become a pleasure. When we first take up any helpful drill we hate it. It hurts. The muscles are sore. We are tired and we want to quit. What we do in this stage cannot be said exactly to be doing us good, but rather getting ready to do us good. The real good comes only with time and as the reward of patient self-discipline, and our exercise becomes a joy, and we run in desire to our practice. The flower and fruit of discipline is always joy.

"All beginnings are difficult," says the proverb. And those who refuse to take the exercise they know to be wholesome, for the reason that they are hard and painful, are ignorant of the great law of results. The pleasure that comes from vigor and a clean, strong body is at the top of a high mountain, and it takes stiff climbing to attain it. Or it is an oasis, and between us and it is a hot weary desert to travel.

Discipline, self-mastery, the renunciation of the present desire for the sake of a distant goal, these are not merely religious motives. They are the essentials to everything worthwhile. You can have no intellectual power without them, and without them you cannot have and keep a healthy body.

Unless one is going to overcome his flabbiness, indecision and weakness, he need not look for any abiding pleasure in life. For these defects will fill his body with disease, worm-eat his mind with ignorance and superstition, and soil the dignity of his spirit.

Whatever you do, stick to it. Time and repetition are what count.

THE *RIGHT* TRAINER CAN HELP!

Have you ever "snaked" your kitchen sink, "sweated" your copper water pipes? Have you ever put down your own floor tile or carpet? Painted your own house? Reshingled your roof? Rewired your electricity? The vast majority of us don't do these things. Why not? Because we don't know how. We don't have the knowledge or the experience. It's that simple.

If we did try to do these things, chances are the roof would leak, carpet seams would show, tile would be uneven, pipes would burst, and drains would stay clogged. We would then spend twice as much money on a professional—not only to fix the original problem, but also to repair the damage we caused trying to do it ourselves. Sound familiar?

Don't make this mistake with your body. It's the damnedest thing, but for whatever reason, people tend to value the pipes in their house more than they value the pipes in their bodies. When it comes to our houses, most of us practice excellent preventive maintenance. We understand the dollars and cents of keeping systems in good operating order. And we understand that a professional is often needed to ensure the success of that maintenance. We know how important those copper pipes are, which is why we don't even hesitate to spend $75 an hour on a plumber.

Keep practicing successful preventive maintenance on your house, your yard, and your car. It's prudent and it's responsible, but always put things in perspective. How nice does your house look from the hospital bed after a triple bypass? How concerned are you with your automatic

Bruce Almighty: A Client's Tale

by Bruce Hayes

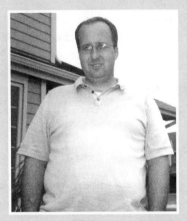

Before

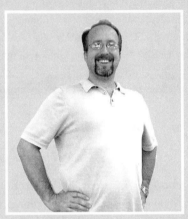

After

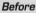

I know what you're thinking: *This guy's "before" picture looks familiar, but his "after" picture isn't anything like the ones I've seen before.* Well, no, I don't have a perfect tan. Nor do I have chiseled abs. And I'd certainly never be caught dead in a Speedo. I'm just a regular person, like you.

My testimonial is quite different from others that usually accompany before and after pictures. First of all, my story began very differently. I didn't wake up one morning and make some major commitment that I was going to spend ninety days or six months dedicated to some exercise and diet regimen. Instead, it began at my gym. My membership was about to expire, and like so many people who belong to gyms, I realized that, aside from the first month or so when I'd been going regularly, I hadn't exactly gotten my money's worth. I decided to talk this over with the owner of the gym. Instead of encouraging me to renew my membership, the owner told me that I shouldn't renew it, that he was tired of people who paid their membership fees and then never came. These people, he said, think they have taken care of the problem by joining a gym, when in fact they are in no better shape than when they began. It should not be surprising that the gym owner and the author of this book are the same person, Marty Tuley.

Marty said that if I was truly serious about losing weight I could start training with him three days a week. After some hesitation and skepticism, I decided to take his advice. I figured I really didn't have much to lose at that point—except a whole lot of weight that is.

Working with a trainer is not just about having someone there to shout at you and push you to do more (although Marty did do a lot of that). For starters, a trainer pushes you to do more while making sure you don't overdo it. Let's be honest: How many times have you lifted weights without guidance, then couldn't walk or move the next day, and subsequently didn't return to the gym? A good trainer is there, in part, to make sure you don't overstrain your muscles.

The most important part of my training experience was the educational aspect. Before training, walking into a weight room was a very daunting experience. Everyone else seemed to know what to do and went about doing it, while I tried to read the diagrams on the machines without being too obvious. But now, thanks to my trainer, when I go into a weight room, I'm neither confused nor intimidated. I feel confident and comfortable and I know what it takes to have a good workout.

I trained with Marty for more than a year. During this time, I did almost no cardiovascular work—no hours on the treadmill, no attempts at jogging. I just lifted weights three times a week for an hour. As for my diet, there was nothing spectacular about it. I did not decrease my caloric intake. I did not stop eating carbs. I just made some sensible adjustments. With Marty's help, I did simple things like educating myself about the fat, carbohydrate, and protein amounts in the food I was eating. If you force yourself to pay attention to what you eat, you quickly realize that you can do a lot better without much effort. Most of us get about 40 percent of our calories from fat, another 50 percent from carbs, especially refined sugars, and if we're lucky, 10 percent from protein. I just set a goal to modify that equation; it became a challenge to see if I could get 40 percent of my calories from protein. Doing that made a huge difference.

I never set a weight-loss goal and when I did lose weight, it snuck up on me. I know that with trendy diets there is the immediate pay-back of pounds lost in a matter of weeks, but this sort of motivation is fleeting. The changes I made in my diet are still there, almost two years after I began this process.

So, the after picture you see above represents a weight loss of about twenty pounds. No one thinks that's impressive enough, spending a year at something and only losing a total of twenty pounds. I couldn't disagree more. I have gone from being clinically obese to being moderately overweight. It won't surprise me if in another year I have reached my ideal body weight. Better than that, though, is that the net loss of twenty pounds is deceptive. Not only is my waist-line significantly slimmer, my muscles are much more developed, which means a higher percentage of my weight is muscle. Changing my metabolism through consistent exercise and exertion has made a huge difference. I am physically stronger than a lot of people that might look more "fit" on the surface.

While it's true that I won't be appearing on the cover of *Muscle & Fitness* any time soon, I don't care. What's important to me is that I can play with my kids without thinking up excuses to stop playing. I can run with them, bike with them, and play sports with them, and that feels wonderful. Also, this past summer I reached the summit of a mountain in Utah—a goal I'd set for myself several years earlier. The goal seemed absurd when I'd set it; this hike is more than twenty miles round trip and takes you from an elevation of 7,200 feet to the summit elevation of almost 12,000 feet. I can't tell you how good it felt when I reached the summit, leaving behind other hikers who seemed fitter than me. I was on top of the world. Still, I won't make the cover of any hiking magazine, but the experience was so exhila-rating that next year I'm going to Colorado to climb an even taller mountain!

If you are still not impressed with my results after a year of train-ing, that's okay. To me, my transformation was miraculous and, more important, it's lasting and ongoing. Maybe someday I'll become a personal trainer. After all, I've had an excellent teacher. In the mean-time, I won't quit my day job, but I *will* continue to work out. . . .

sprinkler system when you're going under the knife to have a tumor removed from your colon? How important is the oil change in your car after a massive stroke? You and your body **must** be NUMBER ONE on your preventive maintenance list!

Okay, you're ready to move yourself up the old priority list. Great! But don't make this common mistake: Don't assume that a $25 a month gym membership automatically vaults you up the list. And don't assume that because you ran down to the nearest sporting-goods store, and some sharp, slick salesman outfitted your house like you're training for the Olympics, that you've moved up the priority list either. After all, you've got tools in your garage, mister, but you're no plumber!

Because we don't know any better, the vast majority of people think personal trainers write exercise programs. They give clients a list of exercises to do, they follow them through the workout counting repetitions, and sometimes correcting form. Unfortunately, this is an accurate description of a lot of personal trainers. However, if this is your trainer and you're paying for it, fire him or her! This is not personal training.

You don't need a babysitter—you need an expert. Or maybe you're one of those people who think you don't need a trainer. I run into these guys daily (and I stress "guys"). For whatever reason, testosterone, ego, or stupidity, guys just can't accept that they could benefit from a knowledgeable trainer. Their loss. You can lead a horse to water, but you can't make him drink.

Think of it like this: the greatest athletes in the world, regardless of sport, have a coach. Michael Jordan is almost, without question, the greatest basketball player to have ever played the game. But he never played the game without a coach. A trainer is a coach—someone who can continue to instruct, teach, provide feedback, and maybe most important, motivate.

So how does a personal trainer figure into the GOYA program? Good question. I have presented an exercise program that is first and foremost designed to get you in the habit of regular exercise. I want you to first realize that a program of regular exercise must be a weekly habit analogous to brushing your teeth (let's hope you're doing this one daily), mowing the yard, mopping the floor, and so on.

Bottom line, for the first 125 days of the GOYA program, you don't need a trainer. Truth be told, you don't need a trainer ever on this program. It's not an exercise program designed to necessarily give you a "six pack," a job as a runway model, or a spot on the next USA Olympic Team. It's designed to create a healthy habit that will enhance—and possibly extend—your life.

But, if at some point you want to take your fitness to another level or create an admirable physique, then using a qualified personal trainer is your next step. The tricky part is finding and hiring a quality personal trainer.

Trust me; despite the apparent plethora of trainers, knowledgeable and experienced trainers are few and far between. There are boatloads of college-educated, certified trainers out there who neither understand nor have any real experience in actually developing, instructing, or properly motivating clients.

What's the biggest problem with the vast majority of personal trainers out there? Lack of experience. They've got college degrees, certifications, and beer bellies! Here's your checklist for identifying a quality, knowledgeable personal trainer.

Certifications. They're a dime a dozen. Certifications (of which there are multitudes) are not completely worthless, but many come close. Some certifications can be obtained over the Internet, while others may require attendance at a weekend seminar or testing site. Some certification courses cost fifty bucks and some cost a whole lot more. A few are actually challenging and require real study time, but too many others are just plain easy.

Obviously, I put very little stock in certifications. That's because some of the best personal trainers I've known didn't have certifications (just years of experience working out themselves) and some of the worst were the most heavily certified. How can this be? Let me give you an example: Most trainers (certified or not) know that a standing barbell curl is a biceps exercise. Some know that if the elbows move forward during this exercise, the anterior deltoid becomes involved and increased stress is placed on the long head of the bicep, which changes the emphasis of the load and possibly increases the risk of shoulder injury. A few know that hand placement, the type of bar used, the body position, and so on all change the action of the muscle, area of emphasis, and even the reason for a particular exercise selection. Very few know what commands to give during the actual exercise and what cues a client needs to hear in order to optimize the movement. And very, very few know how to properly motivate and encourage clients in exercise all together. In short, certifications show an interest, but factored alone they are not an accurate means of assessing how qualified or how knowledgeable a trainer will be.

A final note: The personal training industry is currently in the midst of a substantial change regarding certifications. There has been a major push from both within the industry and corresponding industries to standardize and accredit personal training certifications. It is the inevitable consequence of an industry that has grown so rapidly. When all is said and done, it will hopefully result in more competent, more qualified, and more experienced personal trainers.

College degree. In my opinion, a college degree is more valuable than a certification. At least you know that the trainer spent four years (instead of a weekend) completing it! But here's the thing . . . as a former club owner, I can tell you that most college graduates with a relative degree such as kinesiology or exercise physiology, don't practice what they studied. Without practical application, who cares if they can tell you where the insertion point of the biceps is located, you just want to get in better shape. Be wary of trainers with a lot of college time and little exercise time.

Experience. As far as I'm concerned, experience is what it's all about. I'm not talking about experience training clients (though that's not bad), but experience training themselves! Would you hire a mechanic who doesn't work on his own car? I have heard some trainers argue that potential clients shouldn't consider their (the trainer's) own physical conditioning. The only thing that should matter is their knowledge, education, and experience. Wrong! Would you hire a lawyer who's practicing from inside San Quentin State Prison?

Here's the profile you're looking for in a GOOD personal trainer:

He or she should be at least twenty-six or twenty-eight years old. Any younger and they just haven't had time to make enough trips around the block.

He or she should have a college degree and/or accredited certification. If nothing else, it shows interest.

Look for a trainer with a story about how fitness has changed his or her life. These are the people with passion. Passion can't be taught or bought.

Choose someone you like. You will ultimately have a very intimate relationship with your trainer. It's natural. Find someone with a personality that you're naturally drawn to.

Pick someone with a solid, successful, existing clientele—ask for references.

I have been exercising religiously for *twenty* years! I started at the ripe old age of fifteen and never looked back. I literally started and never stopped. For twenty years I have been a walking, talking exercise experiment. I have tried every program, every exercise, and every technique. I have read, researched, and/or tried every possible combination of protein, carbohydrates, and fat, and I have experimented with every legitimate supplement offered. If I were a lab rat, I'd be retired with a bronze star!

My point? I am still learning! I am still discussing, and I am still experimenting. I don't know it all, and I never will. The learning process never stops—ever. That's not a bad thing. That's the best thing! Enjoy.

A LEANING BUILDING IS A FALLING BUILDING

Poor posture must be contagious because everyone appears to be catching it! You're doing it, and you don't even realize it. I can almost guarantee it. Time to take the kink out—for God's sake, man, stand up!

You're going to be in a lot of fights during your life, but you've never had an opponent like this one. This opponent won't wear out. And if you want a lesson in consistency, look no further. Day in, day out, this guy never stops and never lets up. The painful reality of this fight is: ultimately you will lose. All right, you know what you're up against. But we're not going down easy. We're going down reaching for the ropes. Warriors wouldn't do it any other way.

Gravity is a bitch. From the get-go, we fight it. First, nothing, then slowly we begin to win some battles. We roll over, sit up, and soon thereafter, crawl. One year into this raging war, we take our first significant victory . . . we stand and walk. For the first twenty years or so, we do really well. And most of us don't even realize the war is still raging. Our opponent seems almost nonexistent. But at about twenty-five years old (sometimes earlier, sometimes later), we start losing. Not because we couldn't still win, or at the very least hold our own, but because we become lazy. We allow gravity to begin winning, and we don't even know it.

Stand in front of a full-length mirror. Relax. Stand just as you would if you weren't thinking about it. Now turn your head and take a good long look. Yuck! You've got more kinks than Shirley Temple on a hot, humid summer day! Let's fix this problem.

First, start being aware of your posture; you'll have to make a conscious effort. It just won't take care of itself. Try to catch yourself slumping. If you spend a lot of time at a desk (and many of us do), don't hunch. Even while seated and working, your lower back should have a slight arch, your shoulders should be pulled back and your chest up.

Want to do something really neat? Take a therapy exercise ball to work and use it as a chair. Just make sure it's properly inflated and the right height. Because a therapy ball doesn't have a back or arm rests, your trunk muscles (abdominals and lower back) are forced to compensate. Start slow, maybe an hour or two, and gradually increase the time you spend on the ball, weaning yourself off that old office chair.

Yeah, you'll get some looks and probably be the center of conversation at the water hole for a while. So what! It's a small price to pay for living a longer, healthier, and more enjoyable life.

You'll go through this world one time. Do it with your head high, shoulders back, and chest up. Do it with pride! Look every obstacle and every opportunity straight in the eye.

WHAT HAPPENS AFTER THE FOURTH MONTH?

Good question. You've followed the plan. You've been disciplined and dedicated. But you've finished your fourth month. Where do you go from here? You tell me.

Where did you go when you finished high school? College, maybe? What about after your wedding? Or after the birth of your first child? Where did you go after those events? You went on. That's where.

You went on with your life. You didn't stop learning after you finished school. You continued your education in the field. You gained valuable experience, all the while applying what new knowledge you gained.

You became a parent when you had your child, but you didn't know
all there was to parenting. You continued learning and you continued
expanding your parenting skills.

You've done the same thing with your marriage. Is there a book out
there that will take you step by step from the wedding day to the day
death takes your partner in life. Of course not. The learning process of
creating a successful marriage never stops (if it is to be successful), and
living the health and fitness lifestyle is no different.

I'd love to tell you the GOYA program is all you'll need for the rest of
your life. But more than likely it isn't. You must keep learning about
health and fitness. New information comes to light every single day.
However, there is a BIG difference between being a learner and being a
searcher.

Searchers think the one pill, the one routine, the one piece of equipment is right around the corner. So they search endlessly and tirelessly
for the "golden fleece" of fitness. This is an empty, unfulfilling search
that is never satisfied. A thirst never quenched.

Learners evaluate. They listen. They experiment, but they never abandon the basics. They understand that expanded learning is first and foremost dependent on the knowledge and application of the basics. You
must have a solid foundation, before you ever start building your house.

I have four rules for you from here forward:

1. Exercise

2. Learn

3. Apply

4. ENJOY THE JOURNEY!

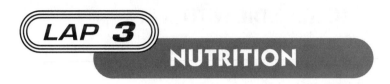

LAP 3 — NUTRITION

What's more important, exercise or nutrition? It's an excellent and an interesting question. If you believe the crap the media and the weight-loss industry has been spoon-feeding you for the last twenty or so years, then like a lot of people (most people) you've been brainwashed into believing that obesity is simply a matter of dieting. Eating specific foods and following a specific plan is all that's necessary to achieve that "body" you've always dreamed about.

Nutrition is key. It is. But, nutrition is not about "points," pills, supplements, high-fat, low-carb, no sugar, fat-blockers, carb-blockers, or a thousand other SCAMS! Oh, you can do any and all of the above; maybe you have. You're also probably fat again, probably even fatter than before you started whatever miraculous weight-loss remedy you last attempted. You've been hoping and wishing for the "magic, eating plan," haven't you? Well as my Uncle Jim is so fond of saying, **"Wish in one hand, shit in the other, and see which one piles up first!"**

Proper nutrition is absolutely essential to your health and fitness success. Make no mistake about it. But nutrition is a component of your success, not the primary or the only mechanism of your success. If you believe nutrition alone will solve your weight issues, you will be fat again. More than likely, you'll be even fatter than before and will live a miserable life of weight loss, weight gain, weight loss, and weight gain. For all the diets you'll try over your life, you'll only have one thing to show for your endeavors. You'll be fatter. I can almost guarantee it.

It's a shitty message. I know it may have just knocked the wind out of your sails but we, YOU, must start with the truth. Because no matter how bitter the pill, if you're going to succeed, this is one you're just going to have to swallow. You want to stick your head back in the sand, I know. It's easier and it's safer. But it's also prolonging the inevitable. The longer you hide from the truth, the longer you'll be mired and stuck in your illusion of success and the less time you'll have to truly enjoy the fruits of what *real* health and fitness success can deliver.

DIET . . . DIE WITH A "T"

Don't do it. Don't buy into any one eating plan or one eating philosophy. They do not work, at least not long term. Why? You will get bored. You will get tired. You will get so sick of the same foods and formats day after day that you will eventually "snap."

Initially, you won't snap hard. You'll just deviate a little, telling yourself that tomorrow you'll get back on track. And you probably will, but that snap will come back. Quicker than the last time. Each time your snap comes back sooner, until eventually, you stay snapped.

Once you stay snapped you enter into the realm of the "yo-yo" dieter. What a wonderful, unfulfilling world this is. This is the world where you bounce from fad diet to fad diet to fad diet. Each time losing weight, gaining more weight, losing more weight, gaining more weight, and continuing to spiral down emotionally, physically, and psychologically, until you ultimately see yourself as a complete failure. You're not a failure, but you are making the wrong choices for the wrong reasons.

Don't be lazy! You are not a failure, but you are being lazy. Quit being lazy! Quit looking for the quick fix! It doesn't exist. It never has and it never will. Success in anything is hard. It is supposed to be. If you want to have success, you'll have to work and work hard. Hard work is what separates the winners from the losers. Losers look for shortcuts and quick fixes because that's easy. Losers buy the "Hollywood Diet"! Oh, did I step on your toes? You bought the Hollywood Miracle Diet? Then your toes should be stepped on! You're lazy! Winners recognize success is hard, very hard. I am reminded of a movie dialogue, which stuck with me from the moment I heard it. See if you remember this on-screen exchange:

"I just didn't think it would be this hard."

"It's supposed to be hard. It's the hard that makes it great!"

This dialogue between the characters played by Tom Hanks and Geena Davis is excerpted from the movie *A League of Their Own*. The point is obvious. Winners work hard! There are exceptions, of course, but the vast majority of truly successful people, regardless of goal, worked plain ole hard. Don't think they didn't. If you're one of those people who think success is largely luck, get out of my way. You're slowing me down!

Most diets don't work for the same reason health clubs don't work. They fail to educate the customer. You cannot drink and eat the same

Three Fad Diets That Should Make You Go *Hmmm* . . .

The Grapefruit Diet

Ah, yes, the infamous means to thin through citrus. My dad actually did this one, and it worked; he lost weight. He also almost died and looked like he'd been stranded on a deserted island for five years! But he lost weight! Oh, and yes, then gained it all back, plus some. Sound familiar?

Pick a food. Any food. Broccoli, deviled eggs, pretzels, vanilla ice cream, TREE BARK! Eat any one food day in and day out, nothing else, and you will lose weight. It isn't brain surgery. It's called starvation! Prisoners of war experience the same results.

The 24- & 48-Hour Hollywood Miracle Diet

I just loved this one. Some orange concoction bottled and sold as a weekend remedy for taking off 10 to 12 pounds just in time for a wedding, a walk down the red carpet, or a funeral (maybe your own). Are you kidding me? The Hollywood Diet's message . . . three delicious drinks a day in place of your meals.

I never bothered to even look at the label on this product, nor did I even think about trying it for curiosity's sake. It doesn't take a genius to figure out that drinking a liquid in place of meals is going to result in some weight loss. It's probably also going to result in a lot of trips to the bathroom and a very clean, shiny colon. So if your colon is going to be on display, here's your baby.

The Atkins Diet

I just wouldn't be doing my job if I didn't address the current, frenzied, low-carbohydrate mania launched by an obscure book written and published more than thirty years ago. The Atkins Diet has changed everything.

The Atkins Diet is not one of my favorites. In fact, I don't endorse it at all. Will it work? Will you lose weight with its application? Yes. However, in my mind, the more important questions are will you keep it off, and, if you do, will you be happier and healthier for it? Probably not.

There is absolutely nothing wrong with complex carbohydrates— brown rice, sweet potatoes, yams, oatmeal, and grits. Complex carbohydrates are naturally occurring nutrients that provide your body, your engine, and your machine with a fuel source. You need complex carbohydrates to power you through your day. There is something wrong, however, with processed and simple carbohydrates such as pasta, white bread, potatoes (in all their forms), and refined sugar. You don't need refined, processed, and bleached carbohydrates that will do little more than spike your insulin levels (not a good thing) and result in unwanted and unneeded fat storage. So, don't cut complex carbohydrates out of your diet, but do cut out white breads, pastas, and refined sugars.

things day in and day out. At some point you have to learn to effectively choose and prepare food. If you don't, you will fail. It's inevitable. You can learn to make the right food choices. You can learn to properly prepare food. You can learn the value of certain foods and nutrients. You can learn when to eat them, how and why. But you won't, if you don't.

SACRIFICE OF THE SCALE

Americans, stop weighing yourself! Have you noticed it isn't doing any good? In case you aren't aware, you're fatter! Want the bad news? It's only going to get worse if you don't make some adjustments.

Remember all those mornings you've woken up, made your way to the bathroom like some giant sloth, pulled your carcass up on some medieval torture device called a scale, looked down with bewilderment because the numbers do nothing but go up!

"How could this be? I skipped two meals yesterday and sat in the sauna for thirty minutes?!" you exclaim.

Good job! How'd that sauna feel? Soothing? Felt like you shed a few pounds? You didn't. Sorry to break it to you. You don't lose fat in a sauna; you lose water. Not a good thing, when you consider that your body is about 70 percent water. Oh, and those meals you skipped? That caused your metabolism to slow down even more. So now you look like a giant raisin, and you have the metabolism of a turtle! Nice combo.

And now (despite your efforts) that number you're so scared of, that device you are a slave to, that mechanical mass of springs and gears that measures the amount of pull the earth's gravity has on your mass, will tell you how you feel, how your day will go, and overall make you feel like crap! Because tomorrow, you'll be heavier. Well, screw that!

I'm going to give you permission to do something you've always secretly wanted to do. Something you've probably dreamed of doing. DESTROY YOUR SCALE! Have some fun. Don't just throw it in the garbage. After the years of abuse you've suffered, it's got it coming.

Go out to the garage and grab the biggest, heaviest hammer you can find. This is actually going to be a workout. This is your first step to getting off your ass, and you will burn 200–400 calories, depending on the intensity. You're going to smash, bash, and batter that scale for twenty minutes! I mean let it have it. Don't hold back. It's been a long frustrating journey, but now it's over.

You've decided you will no longer be a slave to a scale. You will no longer care how much you weigh. Besides, if you lived on Mars, you'd weigh approximately one-fourth of what you do on earth. Would that make you feel better? Should it? Of course not!

20 SIMPLE STEPS TO EATING RIGHT

So now you know what you shouldn't be doing as far as nutrition goes. Diets? Forget it. Focusing solely on your weight? I spit on the scale. So what should you be doing? Well, funny you should ask. I've compiled a list of twenty very simple things you can do to eat more healthfully. I'm not going to go into a big song and dance about why they work; they just do. Trust me. Follow these steps and you'll look better, and more important, you'll feel better.

1. Drink water. Lots of water. Your body is about 70 percent water. Need I say more? Every meal, every time you eat, you drink water.

"But pop tastes better," you say.

#$%@ pop! Your body isn't 70 percent pop! Have one now and then, but pop is not to be your liquid of choice with the majority of your meals. When you do have a pop, it's got to be diet. No exceptions.

"But I don't like the aftertaste."

Fine. Maybe you'd rather go blind as a result of your impending type 2 diabetes? Choices, my friend, choices.

2. Eat breakfast. It ain't a Cinnabon and it ain't Fruit Loops. You just slept six to eight hours—you have to put some quality gas in the tank. Don't skip breakfast. Instead, think complex carbs, like oatmeal or grits, and protein, like egg whites.

3. Eat a minimum of four small meals a day and preferably six! Yes, *six*! And don't tell me you don't have time. Warriors don't make excuses. Up until now you've had all the time in the world to sit on your ass, eat the wrong foods, and not exercise. Since you're not doing that, you've got time to do all the right things. Eating smaller, more frequent meals is one of them.

4. Every time you eat, eat with balance in mind. There are really just three things to be aware of: your intake of lean meat; your intake of breads, pastas, and/or grains; and your intake of vegetables. Making healthy selections within these three groups of food and preparing your dishes wisely are two important steps. Then, control your portions. A very simple and effective way to control your portions is to use the palm of your hand as a guide. Every time you eat, keep your portions of these three foods limited to the size of your palm.

5. Quit worrying about fats. Has it done you any good? Don't necessarily reduce your fats; instead up your lean protein.

6. If you're still counting calories, QUIT! It's a pain in the ass, and it's teaching you nothing. Don't worry about calories; worry about making better food choices.

7. Buy low-fat and low-calorie foods at every opportunity. No, they won't taste the same. But you may live longer and better. That's not a bad tradeoff.

8. In general, quit eating red meat. Go ahead and have red meat once a week, but only *once a week*. From here on out, it's fish and other seafood, chicken, turkey, and egg whites. When you do eat red meat, grill it. (Foods tend to be leaner and meaner when grilled, since a lot of the fat simply melts off.)

9. Significantly cut down on your pasta and breads! Americans eat way—and I mean *way*—too much pasta and bread. "What about whole-wheat breads and pasta?" you ask. "Can't I eat those instead?" Not yet. In the beginning, don't make your changes too complex. Keep them simple. Sure, there's a nutritional difference between white flour and whole-wheat products, but at least in the beginning, make your overall focus on consuming less breads and pastas in general. As you learn and physically progress, you can begin to explore smart bread and pasta choices. For now, avoid nutritional "loopholes" and simply cut back.

10. Quit eating out so often. You eat out because it's convenient and easy. Because you're lazy. On the GOYA program, you can be lazy twice a week, no more. But even when you do go out to eat, make better choices. Almost every restaurant in America will prepare food to your specifications. Tell the chef to use just as little butter and/or oil as necessary. If you get a salad, leave off the cheese and use a low-calorie dressing.

11. Green vegetables are now your best friend. I'm talking broccoli and spinach. These two vegetables are loaded with nutrients. The easiest and the healthiest way to consume them is in a salad. The less you cook them, the better. *Raw* is the word!

12. Eat quality nutrition bars. To eat as often as is necessary, you're going to have to start eating nutrition bars. Not any nutrition bar. We're looking for bars with a minimum of 20 grams of protein and as little sugar as possible.

Experiment to find tastes and brands you like. Even when you do find a bar you like, you'll eventually get tired of it. So keep experimenting. New nutrition bars come out every day.

13. Eat slowly. Take small bites and chew with your mouth closed! Proper digestion starts with chewing. Chew your food. Enjoy it. Taste it. Then swallow it. It's not a race. By eating slower, you'll improve your digestion and fill up sooner. Eating quickly means you'll put more grub away before your stomach has a chance to tell your brain it has had enough.

14. Be wary of sauces. The majority of time, this is the most dangerous aspect of any meal in terms of calories and fats. A large grilled chicken breast has approximately 300 calories, including 57 grams of protein, 0 carbohydrates, and only 6 grams of fat. Douse it in two tablespoons of blue cheese dressing and you add an additional 150 calories, no protein, 1 carbohydrate, and 16 grams of FAT!

15. Don't eat after 8:00 P.M. By this time your metabolism is winding down. Anything you eat is liable to be converted to the wrong type of tissue. When or if you get hungry after 8:00 P.M., grab a large bottle of water and drink.

16. Quit eating junk! You know what I am talking about. Chips, crackers, cookies, and so on. I don't have to tell you they're bad; you know.

17. Quit whining! Suck it up! Eating correctly, eating healthy, eating to live is not (initially) terribly fun. In fact, in the beginning it sucks. That's because for the last ten, the last twenty, the last thirty, or the last forty years, you've been stuffing your face (and consequently your ass) with high-sugar, high-fat, and rich-tasting crap. Both your physiology and your psychology have been shaped by specific types and tastes of food. In short, you're addicted. Breaking the addiction, any addiction, is hard, hard, HARD work. BUT that's also why it is so rewarding.

Hard work and great rewards go hand in hand. Jump off the pity wagon, roll up your sleeves, change your life, and reap the rewards.

18. Don't do it alone. Don't just change your eating habits. Change your boyfriend's, your husband's or wife's, and/or your kid's. Everyone can eat better and everyone can feel better for it!

19. Quit using the word *diet.* You are not on a diet. You are changing your lifestyle. Starting a diet infers that at some point you'll have to stop. Changing your lifestyle is forever.

20. Get off your ass!

SO WHAT EXACTLY CAN I EAT?

I do not believe in laying out a specific, detailed eating plan. Why? Because you don't learn that way. You don't educate yourself about what you're eating and why. You don't learn how to make the right choices for the right reasons. You blindly follow a specific eating routine until you're so bored and tired of eating the same shit, you quit. Been there?

You have to eat better, but you have to learn why. Learning is the key. Once again, read this carefully and remember:

If you don't learn the *whats* and *whys* of why you are stuffing your face with certain foods, you will fail!

I know it sounds pessimistic, but the numbers don't lie. The simple fact is nine out of ten people who start an exercise and/or nutritional program will quit within the first ninety days. If you don't want to be included in that statistic, you'd better have a firm understanding of the above statement.

Okay, basically what we are talking about here are carbohydrates, proteins, and fats. One gram of carbohydrate and one gram of protein both have 4 calories. On the other hand, fat has slightly double that, 9 calories. That's why the "fat scare" occurred in the early 1980s and why for years the message was, "fat bad, carbohydrate good."

My, how things change! Now, the root of all our fat problems stem from overconsumption of carbohydrates, or at least that's what we're being told. Now carbohydrates are to blame, never mind TV, video games, computers, and desk jobs. Now all our obesity problems can be solved by eating bacon and butter. Wrong.

Balance, my friend—balance and moderation. If you take nothing else from this book, take that. Those people who are happiest in life and self have mastered balance and moderation in all aspects of their lives. For long-term, real success, your daily eating must be based on balance and moderation.

The following table contains a partial list of GOYA-approved foods. While I'm not trying to be overly simplistic, I don't want to get too specific. You'll likely eat certain foods that aren't listed in the table. That's okay. For instance, I don't typically recommend bananas, but you'll notice that they are listed as an ingredient in one of the GOYA recipes. So, even though they're not on the list, bananas are okay once in a while. Also, corn is not listed as a GOYA-approved food, but this vegetable will cross your path quite often, and it's okay to eat it from time to time. Occasionally eating non-approved foods is not going to kill you. Remember, however, that the key is to practice balance and moderation. Since strict adherence to a daily eating plan is a surefire way to fail, it's okay to cross the centerline now and then. Occasional screw-ups or making less-than-best choices doesn't mean quit; they mean refocus. It's not all or

GOYA-APPROVED FOODS

Grains

brown rice	oatmeal	whole-grain bread
oat bran	wheat bran	whole-grain pasta

Vegetables

asparagus	cucumbers	peas
beans	eggplant	peppers
broccoli	garlic	spinach
Brussels sprouts	lettuce	squash
cabbage	mushrooms	sweet potatoes
cauliflower	onions	zucchini
celery		

Meat

beef, lean	fish	pork
chicken	lamb	shellfish

Dairy

low-fat cottage cheese	low-fat milk	low-fat yogurt
low-fat/non-fat cheese		

Fruit

apples	cherries	mangos
apricots	dates	peaches
avocados	grapefruits	pears
berries	honeydews	plums
cantaloupes	lemons	pumpkin

Other

egg whites	soy milk	spices
nuts		

nothing folks. After you cross that line, just cross back and stay a little longer.

The preparation of the foods listed in the table is just as important as the foods themselves. Choosing GOYA-approved foods won't do you much good if you smother them in buttery sauces. So, not only do you need to make better choices, but you also have to practice smarter preparation. Nothing complex, just use your "noodle" and apply common sense when preparing your food.

Here's your visual for food consumption. Think steam engine and think coal. Your body is the train, what you put in it is your coal. What you want is an engine that burns constantly. Never let your fire go out. That fire is your metabolism. If the fire goes out, your metabolism slows down. That's a bad thing. Keep your metabolism burning. This is why eating smaller more frequent meals is the best way to lose weight. You're keeping the fire burning and keeping your train rolling.

It's damn hard to eat healthy! That's a fact. I am not going to blow any sunshine up your ass. Cravings and wants will always be there. New clients often ask me, "When will I not want junk food?" The answer: probably never. Hell, who doesn't like a bag of M&Ms? You think I don't have the desire to roll through McDonald's for lunch? Think again. I make a choice. You'll have to make a choice. That's life, my friend.

WHY YOUR GRANDPARENTS WEREN'T FAT

Your grandparents fried everything! They drank coffee with every meal, only knew of one kind of milk—whole—and never exercised. By today's standards they did everything wrong! But their obesity levels were half, if not a fourth, of today's levels. Why?

Your grandparents worked! They worked hard! Six days a week, ten hours a day, and that work was predominantly physical. Your grandparents got off their asses! And, quite frankly, they were just plain tougher. They didn't have a scientific name for every ache and pain, and most important, they didn't go seeking them out.

Your grandparents shouldered a lot of the blame and took responsibility for a lot in their lives. In fact, they took responsibility for everything in their lives! Your grandparents believed that, for the most part, they controlled their destiny. And they were unwilling to concede any less.

Have You Ever Seen a Fat Carnivore?

You're going to have to eat more protein. It's that simple. The majority of us just don't consume enough quality low-fat protein. Why? There are several reasons.

First, preparing a protein meal typically takes a little longer than boiling some pasta and heating up sauce. So most of us are just being a little lazy. With a little more planning, you'd have the time to prepare a meal with more protein in it. You're just choosing not to. Don't do this. You're choosing to be fat and lazy. How about choosing to be healthier and happier? Novel concept, huh?

Second, you think eating meat is going to be more expensive. Yeah, chicken costs more than pasta. No question. But, you're thinking short term, wayyyyyy too short-term. Because brother, sister, you're running a tab!

That money you're saving now, it isn't worth it. It's costing you years! Years of quality life. Years of time spent with your family. Years of time spent doing what you love. They don't print enough money to cover those items. Besides, with a little planning and some attentive shopping, you won't even notice the dollar difference.

Third, some people just don't like meat. No problem, you just have to find another way to get your protein. This is where supplements come in handy. Probably the simplest, easiest way to get protein is with a protein powder. Pick a flavor, any flavor—the multitude of choices out there is amazing. Experiment to find one you like. You're looking for a product with 20 to 30 grams of high-quality whey protein per serving and little or no sugar. If you don't have a blender, get one. There is no easier, more convenient way to prepare and consume a meal.

Fourth, you're still using the U.S.D.A. Food Pyramid, which recommends an inadequate amount of protein. The United States is a great country. However, unfortunately, because of its size and bureaucracy, it's sometimes a little behind in the latest research. The U.S.D.A. Food Pyramid isn't necessarily bad; it's just not the best. And baby, you deserve the best.

Fifth, for whatever reason, you haven't heard of "the incredible, edible egg"! Eggs are the most easily digested, assimilated, and naturally occurring protein source known. Your body loves them. Omelets are awesome. (Try Lana's Egg Whites; visit www.lanaseggwhites.com.) Non-fat cheese, broccoli, mushrooms, tomatoes, and turkey; what a combo! Just two rules: use a fat-free and calorie-free cooking spray and use only one yolk to every three eggs used.

Now I will be the first to tell you that your grandparents probably weren't "martyrs." It is okay to ask for help, and it is okay to need it. But for the vast majority of us (remember I am talking about the masses in general), we don't need a diagnosis. We don't need a pill. We don't need a fancy word or scientific terminology. The vast majority of us just need to get off our ass!

It is probably your grandparent's physical activity that allowed them to eat and live in the manner they did. Your grandparents didn't eat a lot of processed carbohydrates. The bulk of their nutrition came from protein, fats, and complex carbohydrates. This is by no means a startling revelation. Processed carbohydrates and the eating habits that accompany them are a relatively new phenomenon for human civilization.

Opinions vary, but most experts agree, the influx of processed carbohydrates in our everyday diets coupled with decreased activity is propelling us toward off-the-chart obesity levels. In theory, had we maintained the level of physical activity of our grandparents, we might have transitioned successfully to a diet high in processed carbohydrates. However, whatever the cause, whatever the reason, it's water under the bridge now.

Again, it's an opinion, but many experts agree that humans are not designed or engineered for processed-carbohydrate consumption. We are designed to burn fat and naturally occurring complex carbohydrates as our energy source. It's genetic; our ancestors were designed this way. This is essentially the concept behind the Atkins diet.

However, while I believe this diet may be sound in theory, it is doomed to failure. Why? Because processed carbohydrates are here to stay and desk jobs are here to stay. We just need to learn how to effectively choose carbohydrates, efficiently consume them, and be a little more like our grandparents.

The question is, how do we do this? Here's one suggestion: get with the GOYA program and get off your ass!

WEIGHT LOSS WITHOUT EXERCISE: SAY WHAT?

Forget it! I thought . . . just for a moment, of ending this section with those two first words, simple, clean, and to the point. But then I thought again. Being active in the health and fitness arena for more than twenty years sometimes makes me overlook the obvious. Sometimes, in fact, a lot of times, people just don't know any better. Get ready to know better.

The weight-loss industry is enormous. Billions of dollars are spent annually on products and services designed, developed, and marketed for weight loss. I can prove to you with one statement why 99 percent of these products are trash: You're a citizen of the fattest country in the world, and it's getting worse every day!

You, the consumer, are spending billions of dollars to lose fat, and instead you are getting fatter. I'd start thinking *refund*! And you were worried you were wasting your money in the stock market. The weight-loss industry has it made. They keep turning out products to make you thin. You keep buying them as fast as they hit the shelves. Then you continue to get fatter and continue to buy weight-loss products. The weight-loss industry isn't just penetrating the market; they appear to be building and developing it!

SUPPLEMENTS? SUPPLE*MESS!*

Got an ache or a pain? Do you have a lack of this or a lack of that? Do you have hair where you don't want it? No hair where you need it? Dry cuticles? Low energy or too much energy? Depression? Anxiety? Trouble sleeping? Trouble sleeping too much? High body fat? Low body fat?

Walk into your local health food store and a teenager with spiked hair and acne will try to solve your problem with a pill. That alone should send you rushing for the exit door.

There are some valued uses for supplements. There are some valued products and companies. But unfortunately, there is a whole lot of snake oil on the market with all sorts of outrageous claims accompanying them. Here's my opinion on the good, the not-so-good, and the just plain ugly of supplements.

The Good

Whey protein. Simple, effective, and the most overlooked and underutilized nutritional aspect of the American diet; two servings daily (mid-morning and mid-afternoon) as part of a balanced diet.

MRPs (meal replacement powders). A close second, and I mean close.

It just depends on your individual needs. In today's society, our biggest obstacle to eating correctly is probably time; hence, the success of fast FAT food.

MRPs allow you to quickly, efficiently, and tastefully consume a balanced meal. For a lot of people, they provide a simple means of getting that all-important breakfast, but they're an equally effective lunch.

Multivitamin/mineral. Simple, inexpensive, and effective. As my wife says, "Better to have expensive urine, than a cheap body."

The Not-So-Good

Creatine. Creatine has dominated supplement talk for several years now, and it is not without merit for performance athletes, bodybuilders, and weight lifters. However, I liken creatine to icing on the cake. For the Average Joe, that guy or gal out there just looking to get in better shape, this supplement is probably a waste of money.

Glutamine. I throw this one in with creatine. It has some merit for athletes, but I just don't think it's a supplement for the majority of us. This again, is an example of icing on the cake. Forget about the icing—we're still working on the cake itself.

Branched chain amino acids. These amino acids are considered essential because we cannot survive without them in our daily diet. They're instrumental in the maintenance of muscle tissue, help prevent muscle protein breakdown during exercise, and may also preserve muscle stores of glycogen (stored carbohydrates). All that being said, their role as a necessary supplement is probably overemphasized. As with a lot of supplements, their overall impact is so slight that their use should probably be limited to those people who are pushing the envelope of their physical abilities.

The Plain Ugly

Fat burners. Bunk! I am not for fat burners. I don't like the idea of stimulants. Natural or not, they make me uneasy and they make you lazy. Why take a pill to make your heart beat faster? Isn't that what exercise is for? If you really want to give your heart a little jolt before a workout, drink a cup of coffee.

Effective supplementation is not complicated. Most of us make it complicated by being searchers. Remember what I said earlier? If you're a searcher, you're a slacker. Searchers are looking for the answer to health and fitness in a bottle. Warriors know there is no such thing.

What You Need

You'll need three supplements and three only with the GOYA program.

1. **Whey protein.** For beginners or veterans, this is your first and most important supplement purchase.

2. **MRPs.** If you find it either too difficult or simply impossible to eat a balanced breakfast, lunch, and/or dinner, then you'll need an MRP product. Be wary of utilizing MRPs for mid-morning, mid-afternoon, or late-evening snacks (mini-meals), unless you're using a product with few or no carbohydrates. Use MRPs for your primary meals and think protein, vegetables, and/or nuts for the in-between food sessions.

There are no shortages of manufacturers. Don't think of this as an additional expense to your budget, since you'll be using the product as a meal replacement. MRP is now part of your grocery list.

Here's a simple, tasty recipe for a delicious MRP:

1 serving of vanilla MRP

8 ounces skim milk or water

½ banana

1 cup ice

Combine ingredients in blender, and blend until smooth. Enjoy!

---

3. **A quality multivitamin/mineral.**

LAP **1**

+ LAP **2**

+ LAP **3**
_____

A Better YOU

All right, let's put it all together.

You started practicing Lap One before you starting exercising. Good. You practiced Lap One for four weeks. You started your conditioning program with the first step virtually everybody ignores—you started by first conditioning your mind.

Lap One is critical to your long-term success. Why? Because everyone in the world starts an exercise program with the physical, and virtually everyone who starts fails. They fail because, ultimately, they lose the battle in their minds, not in their bodies. Don't stop practicing the principles of Lap One. Indeed, expand upon them. Continue to exercise your mind as rigorously as you exercise your body.

In Lap Two you started exercising with one thirty-minute workout a week. Clearly not enough, and everyone knows that. But what's the point of starting with three or even five workouts a week if you fail in a month or even six months?

Remember, this isn't about time. This isn't a three-month, six-month, or one-year program; this is the program for life. Results will come. Besides, if for the last ten years you've done NOTHING, then one day a week of regular exercise is a good start. No, it's a *great* start!

Your neighbor may initially laugh at your exercise program. Visit him or her in five years. In five years, your neighbor's been on no less than five exercise programs, as many diets, has been a member of two health clubs, and is 10–20 pounds heavier! Now who's laughing?

Nutrition is a BIG part of the battle. But that doesn't necessarily mean it needs to encompass 400 pages of reading. Nor does it need to be definitive, regimented, or prescribed. The vast majority of us just need to make better decisions, like the ones outlined in Lap Three.

And don't play stupid! You know, generally, what's good and bad; you just choose to ignore your own instincts. Don't follow a stringent diet. Make better choices. Follow the simple rules in Lap Three. Just those little "tidbits" will have a huge impact on your conditioning.

The GOYA program is not intended to be an end-all. It could be. I firmly believe you could perform this simple routine your entire life, and live much better and richer for it. But the keys to advancing your program lie in Lap One.

This is a journey. You know the path. The means, pace, and distance are now fully in your control.

Time to don your armor, sharpen your blade, and mount your trusty steed. The war is raging. Enjoy the battle.

LAST CHANCE

WE'VE FINALLY RECOGNIZED THE MAGNITUDE of the obesity epidemic with the adult population. Good. We've finally acknowledged that obesity will soon be the number-one killer of adults, surpassing the long-standing and reigning champ, cigarettes. Whether this knowledge and admission will ultimately lead to a society that eats better and exercises regularly remains to be seen. But it's a start. However, starting from the top down may prove an effort in futility if we don't also address and understand that the even bigger obesity time bomb is still there, quietly ticking. Will we diffuse this bomb in time?

Junior's Not So Junior-sized

One of the most troubling stats with regard to obesity in this country has manifested in our youth. Our kids are fat! *REAL* fat. And we'd better figure out why, real quick. Their future, and ours, depends on it!

Take a look at the stats:

- The number of overweight children has doubled in the last two to three decades.

- 30 percent of children and teens are overweight and the number is rising.

- 11 percent of preschool children are considered obese.

- 12.6 percent of thirteen-year-old boys are overweight.

- 10.8 percent of thirteen-year-old girls are overweight.
- 13.9 percent of fifteen-year-old boys are overweight.
- 15.1 percent of fifteen-year-old girls are overweight.
- One in three children born in 2000 will develop type 2 diabetes.
- Diabetes will reduce their life expectancy by seventeen to twenty-seven years.
- An overweight child has a 70 percent chance of being an obese adult.
- When one parent is obese, there is a 50 percent risk the children will be obese.
- When both parents are obese, there is an 80 percent risk the children will be obese.

Why are our children fat? It's a question being pondered, debated, and researched in many circles. The answer often seems complicated and intricate. There have been numerous studies and investigations, some complete and many ongoing with many more yet to come. The academics and lab boys will be studying this problem to death. And all the while our kids will get fatter, get teased, develop type 2 diabetes, and die young. Well, I'm not willing to wait. Let's just look at the facts and apply a little common sense.

Have you been to school with your kids lately? Have you eaten lunch with them? Did you happen to notice that our schools no longer have kitchens and cooks? They don't have to. Everything served is processed, precooked, and loaded with low-quality carbohydrates, sugar, fat, and little or no protein. With this menu we don't need kitchens or cooks, just microwaves and servers, and that's exactly what we've got.

I don't think you need a Ph.D. to recognize that today's school lunches have simply become "fast food." Logistics, economics, and politics have all had a hand in turning our school lunch program, which serves 27 million meals daily, into an assembly line of junk food; simple to store and easy to prepare. Our children's nutrition has taken a backseat to needs of the bureaucracy.

Okay, we've got nutritionally bad school lunches. But, in my opinion, school lunches are the least of our problems. Let's face it, that's only one hour and one meal in a twenty-four-hour day. What about the other twenty-three hours?

Did you know physical education (PE) is not a daily part of most school curricula? Only 8 percent of today's elementary schools provide daily physical activity. Exercise is not a part of life for today's youth. Nearly half of today's youth between the ages of twelve and twenty-one are not vigorously active on a regular basis. In most school systems, PE is now only a part of the WEEKLY curriculum. Most kids have PE once a week, and a lot of kids aren't even getting that! Poor school lunches and no daily PE, hmmmmmm . . . I wonder why we have an obesity epidemic among children? Please. Think! We don't need five years of studies, research, and millions of tax dollars to figure this problem out. Organizations like PE4Life are already taking up the fight.

PE4Life is a non-profit organization bent on the reestablishment of quality routine physical education at all levels in our public schools. Their organizational goals are:

- Raise awareness about the physical inactivity levels of America's youth and the state of physical education across the nation.

- Promote the need for reforming educational policy to include mandatory daily physical education classes for children in grades K–12.

- Promote model quality physical education programs in every state.

- Empower physical educators, parents, and community leaders to become advocates for quality daily physical education.

- Stimulate private and public funding for quality physical education.

For more information on this fabulous organization, or to learn how you can be involved and make a difference, visit www.PE4life. com.

PE isn't alone; outside recess has followed a similar diminishing role in the typical school day. Recess has become synonymous with computer games. Is that the kids' fault? Of course not. Given the option, most kids would pick computer games over kickball. It's easier and more convenient. But it's not necessarily right, healthy, or in the child's best interest.

Lawyers and fear-mongers have managed to all but shut down outside recesses in an effort to keep our children safe. Ironic isn't it. We no longer allow kids recess to protect them from physical harm and, in doing so, create an epidemic of obesity that will haunt them through most of their lives. Well-intentioned parents and money-hungry lawyers have sacrificed bruises, scrapes, and bumps for depression, low self-esteem, type 2 diabetes, high blood pressure, heart disease, cancer, joint problems, and sleep disorders, to name a few.

When I was a kid (jeez, I sound like my father), there would be days with a foot of snow on the ground but we still went outside for recess. In fact, we didn't have the option not to. Teachers wanted a break, and we had energy that needed to be used. We went outside. We got bundled up. We got cold. We got wet. And we sometimes caught colds. But we weren't fat!

After school isn't much better, despite what appears to be a growing number of venues for childhood athletics (Little League soccer, football, baseball, and so on). The fact is, the numbers say that just isn't so. 61.5 percent of kids between the ages of nine and thirteen DO NOT participate in any organized physical activity. Why? Lack of funding has placed public schools in the precarious position of program cuts. The result: either no school-sponsored athletic programs or "pay to play," a system with obvious bias to particular social strata.

But schools and budgets aren't solely to blame. The typical high school senior now graduates with approximately 12,000 hours of class time and 15,000 hours of lying on his or her ass, watching-TV time—can't blame schools for that one. TVs and computers have replaced bicycles and ballparks, all under the watchful, mindful (though sometimes misguided) eye of the parent.

Get your kids out. Let 'em get some scrapes and bruises. Let 'em get dirty. Let 'em get filthy. Protecting our children should always be one of our foremost considerations, but not at the expense of their adult health. It's akin to buying short-term products with long-term credit. How well does that work?

If we are not careful, we are very quickly going to end up with a generation of wimps. Fat wimps! Get your kids off their asses! If you don't, when you are seventy, you may find your kids are not able to take care of you. Instead, you may find yourself taking care of your overweight, asthmatic, high cholesterol, high blood pressure, triple by-pass waiting-to-happen fifty-year-old son or daughter! How does that sound? Oh, but here's the consolation prize, he's the Grand World Champion of Super Combat III!

Fido's Fat!

Take a good long look at your dog. He's fat—and getting fatter! You know how people are always saying that dog owners look like their pets, and vice versa? Next time someone tells you that you look like your pet don't smile and think it's cute . . . it probably isn't a compliment.

Give us the chance, and we'll screw up almost anything. We take a perfectly good carnivore, molded, and finely tuned by nature and evolution. We pluck it from the wild, confine it to a 20-foot by 20-foot backyard, change its diet from meat to processed carbohydrates (sound familiar?), and give it only enough mental stimulus to keep it from going crazy, but at the same time reward lethargic and lazy (we call it, well-mannered) behavior. This isn't a pet. It's a vegetable!

Our pets mirror us. They get little or no exercise, and they consume a cheap, low-grade protein with a substantial portion of processed carbohydrates. Ask any veterinarian, and he or she will tell you that obesity and all of the attendant medical disorders stemming from this poor diet are causing an ever-increasing, almost epidemic problem with pets. Throw in asthma and attention deficit disorder (both on the rise with family pets), and soon you won't be able to tell your pet's problems from your neighbor's!

It gets worse. We hire people to exercise our dogs. Although we recognize that our dogs need exercise, we're always too busy, or too lazy, to do it ourselves—so we outsource it. We fail to realize or acknowledge that walking man's best friend is not only in Fido's best interest, but also in our own!

We're fat; our kids are fat, and we drag our dogs along for the ride. Jeez. It's not enough that we are killing ourselves—now we're taking passengers! Fido could be your key. I guarantee that no matter the time of day, or how old Fido is, or even if he's gotten a little overweight and out of shape, he's ready to go for a walk! So, if you won't initially get off your ass for yourself, maybe you can do it for him. Fido's not just your best friend; he's your treadmill with a leash!

Wisdom is knowing what to do next; virtue is doing it.

—David Starr Jordan

CONCLUSION

Wrap It Up, I'll Take It!

DON'T EXERCISE SIMPLY FOR THE SAKE OF EXERCISE. Don't do it to look good in your jeans. Don't do it to get more attention at work or when you're out and about. That's not the point. Looking good in your clothes or garnering more attention from those around you can be enjoyable byproducts of the health and fitness lifestyle, but they cannot be your reason for it.

Start and maintain the health and fitness lifestyle for yourself. Definitely reward yourself. Enjoy the obvious stuff—better-fitting clothes, people taking notice of your physique and improved self-confidence, and so on. The fact is, you're just going to feel a hell of a lot better and everyone's going to know it! Great! But that's only step one. You are on the path; now you must take the journey.

Many people step on the path but then fail to take the journey. They get caught, caught in the narcissistic web that often accompanies physical improvement. You must avoid this web, or if caught, work hard to free yourself. The narcissistic web can lead to a never-ending quest for physical perfection. It can lead to endless cosmetic surgery, eating disorders, and even the ultimate loss . . . fracturing of families.

The narcissistic web can lead to a shell of an existence, a world that revolves around only the physical self. Ultimately this world has no substance. This is a shallow and self-destructive world. People caught in this web ultimately fall off the path altogether having never experienced the journey of fitness and all its accolades.

Having a healthy body is not an end-all. It's a beginning, the beginning of improving every other aspect of your life and the beginning of experiences for which you've only dreamed.

Being physically fit is simply the vehicle that allows you to reach new and exciting destinations. Your physical fitness is the means by which you experience and achieve the *really* important stuff.

Think of it like this: Your car has nothing to do with you. It doesn't define you, it isn't your motivation, it isn't anything! It's a piece of metal that takes you from point A to point B. It is a cog, one of thousands, turning in the complexity of our lives. This cog, like many others, is necessary of course, because the machine of life is dependent on its correct functioning. The more cogs operating correctly in our lives, the richer our lives typically are. But, although we need all of our cogs turning and functioning at optimum levels for the ultimate experience of life, the cogs themselves cannot become our focus.

Your body is a cog, an extremely important cog, but a cog. Hone and tune your cog. Push your cog to its production limits but always remember it is simply a means to enrich our lives.

What is *really* important? Only you can answer that. Only you can determine and decide what will define your existence. But certainly, a critical step is simply to . . . **Get off your ass!**

APPENDIX A

FAQs about GOYA, Health, and Fitness

Q If someone wants to lose weight, isn't cardio more important than weight training?

A. No! Both exercises burn calories, but cardio alone has one major short-coming. It does not build muscle. Building muscle is the key. Muscle requires energy. The more muscle you have, the higher and hotter your "engine" (that is, your metabolism) burns. Weight training builds muscle. Take out a pad and pencil and write this down. A fat cell in your body requires only **TWO** calories a day to maintain itself. A muscle cell requires **THIRTY-EIGHT**! Do you get it?! Let me explain further. The fatter you get, the less you move. The less you move, the less muscle you maintain. The more muscle you lose, the less calories your body requires. In short, the fatter you get, the easier it gets to get FATTER. It's a nasty cycle that you can stop only by moving your ass—and that includes *both* cardio and weight training!

Q Isn't it true that to get rid of my "spare tire," I only have to do crunches and sit-ups?

A. Wrong! Crunches and sit-ups are good abdominal exercises. They strengthen and build the muscles that make up your midsection. They DO NOT burn fat. The body utilizes fat reserves evenly throughout the body. This means that for most of us, the first place we want it off is the last place it actually comes off, because this is where the highest fat stores are located. Your "spare tire" isn't the problem; it is the result of your lifesyle. The problems are those daily trips through the McDonald's drive-thru. The problem is your cushy desk job and its inherent paper pushing. Don't exercise to get rid of your spare tire. Exercise because your life and its quality depend on it; and that will get rid of your "spare tire."

Q **Won't working out with weights make me big?**

A. Have you looked in the mirror lately? No? Walk over and take a look—chances are you're already big. If you don't want to be big, stop doing what you're doing. Apply a little logic here, folks. If sitting on your ass has gotten you to where you are, then getting off your ass and lifting weights isn't going to make it bigger. Lifting weights builds lean muscle. That's not a bad thing. That's exactly what you need. Lean muscle needs energy and energy comes from food and fat stores. You MUST build lean muscle!

Q **When we get older, doesn't our metabolism slow down?**

A. When we age, our metabolism does slow down, but this is primarily due to loss of muscle tissue. Why do we lose muscle tissue as we age? Because instead of moving our asses, we're sitting on them! Stop using age as an excuse for getting fat, and start exercising!

Q **If I stop exercising, will my muscles turn to fat?**

A. Muscle tissue can't turn to fat tissue. It's a physiological impossibility. You can't turn dirt to gold either. Muscle does not turn to fat if you quit exercising, but don't expect it to stick around either. If you don't keep building it, it will break down. Don't think you can build muscle then stop working out and still wow the opposite sex. But why would you quit exercising anyway? Quit thinking "program" and start thinking lifestyle.

Q **Isn't exercise just for the young?**

A. Please. You're never too old. Too stubborn, maybe. Too lazy, probably. Too old, **NEVER!**

Q Should I exercise if I have a bad back?

A. Damn straight! Joints go bad because the supporting musculature gets weak and leaves the joint susceptible to harm. Do you want to avoid an injury or recondition your joints and get some more mileage out of them? Exercise! It's the only way you'll make it to your gray years with mobility, grace, and dignity. If you think your back is bad now, just wait until you're sixty! Start exercising.

Q Aren't there dangers associated with overexercising?

A. Very, very few people actually overexercise. Oh, it's out there. Any activity can become an addiction, ultimately leading to a counterproductive or even destructive behavior. But in a country with an obesity percentage closing in on 70 percent, you probably don't need to worry.

Q Am I fat because I eat carbohydrates?

A. Carbohydrates are not bad. Eating too many carbohydrates, especially refined carbohydrates, is bad. So is sitting on your ass. Carbohydrates are *not* the cause of our obesity epidemic. Carbohydrates were around fifty years ago, a hundred years ago, five thousand years ago. In fact, people ate bread while they were building the pyramids! Do you think the Egyptians were fat? Nah. You're not fat because you eat carbohydrates. You're fat because you've been sitting on your ass. Quit being lazy, and you'll probably quit being fat.

Q Isn't eating healthy foods boring cause there's no variety?

A. News bulletin, folks. Fat people don't eat a wide variety of food either! I get this comment all the time from new clients: "How boring—you eat the same foods everyday." So I ask them to start recording the foods they eat for one week, and lo and behold, what do we discover? They (and you, too) eat the same crap, day in and day out. Yes, you do! It's just your mindset: You think live-long-and-healthy broiled fish is boring but Sonic's die-of-a-massive-coronary pancake on a stick is exciting. Change your mindset.

Q Isn't it true that I'm fat because I have the "fat gene"?

A. Seriously think about this for a second. Why has obesity seemingly just become a problem in our country? What's changed in our society in the last couple of decades? Did a tribe of fat people infiltrate our gene pool? Are obese aliens abducting us one by one and infecting us with other-worldly fat cells? We're fat because we eat more calories than we burn. It's that simple. We don't burn as many calories as our forefathers because our country's workforce is almost entirely sedentary. That's okay and that's not going to change anytime soon. So, one of two things has to happen: we have to start eating a lot less (and I mean A LOT) or we have to start exercising like maniacs. Better yet, how about something between those two extremes. Now, there's an idea: moderation. What a concept.

Q How will I ever make time for exercise with my busy schedule?

A. How do you not? How can you afford not to? Do you think you're saving time? Time for what? Time to fight your impending type 2 diabetes? Time to lay in a hospital bed while a doctor inserts stents in your arteries to keep blood pumping through your clogged pipes? Or maybe you're just saving up time for that exciting ambulance ride you'll be taking right after your massive coronary at age fifty. No time to exercise? Pal, time is all any of us really have.

Q I've got a limited budget, so how can I afford to eat right and exercise?

A. You're not saving any money by not eating right and not exercising. You're simply running a tab! Make no mistake, you *will* pay eventually. And you'll pay heavily! Do you think you can eat crap, sit on your ass, and grow old happily and have a little money saved for retirement? Think again. You're more likely to just grow wider and more miserable, and your savings will go toward your huge doctor bills. Start your health and fitness savings account, now!

Q How long after I'm on the GOYA program will my cravings for sweets go away?

A. Your cravings, your desire for sweets, will never "go away." It is, and has always been, about choices and consequences. Choose wisely.

Q Is the GOYA program enough?

A. This is a good question, but more important, "enough" for what? Will you make the women's Olympic gymnastic team with this program? No. Will you be auditioning for a job as a cover model? I doubt it. The GOYA program is designed to introduce routine and regular activity into your daily life. This program is not going to make you look like Vin Diesel or Jennifer Garner. But, it is a start. It's *enough* for now. I'm showing you the journey. You'll have to pick your destination.

Q How soon can I expect to see physical changes on the GOYA program?

A. Never think or believe that a system will "change" you. A system is a tool. Nothing more. Just because you've got a hoe doesn't mean your garden is free of weeds. The changes you see on the GOYA program will be a direct result of your level of consistency, dedication, and EFFORT. There's no "magic bullet" system. Ultimately, your success or failure at anything resides in you. You'll either decide that your physical fitness is worth changing or you won't. The GOYA program is a damn good hoe, but it requires dedication and willpower. The bottom line: you'll see physical changes when *you decide to.*

Q Can't I just accept my obesity and be one of those jolly fat people?

A. If you really think so, you're kidding yourself. By even considering this, you're wasting your most valuable asset—time. How do I know? Let me ask you this: If I were a genie and offered to make you trim and fit, would you let me do it? Of course you would. If you claim otherwise, you're lying to me, to your friends, and, most important, to yourself. If you simply don't want to do the necessary work and put in the required time to be at an ideal body weight and in good physical shape, just say so. It's okay to say, "I don't want to put in the time or effort to achieve that goal." What's not okay is denying that health and fitness are linked to happiness and thinking that you can be fat and unhealthy and still be happy.

Q With so many health and fitness books on the market, what makes following the advice in *Get Off Your Ass!* my best choice?

A. I'd like to tell you that the GOYA program is the holy grail of fitness and that it will lead this fat country to fitness salvation. But the truth is there are a lot of books out there that offer sound advice and good fitness programs. The biggest obstacle for most people is a lack of consistency. The GOYA program eases you into it—okay, pushes you a bit—into the habit of exercising and making responsible choices, reminding you every step of the way that you can do it if you just get off your ass!

Q To stay fit, shouldn't I participate in exercise activities that I think are fun?

A. This is one of the most destructive fallacies of health and fitness, and I want to "strangle" trainers and so-called experts when I hear them say "find an exercise you think is fun." Trust me, if you think the secret to your health and fitness success is an endless search for "fun" exercise, brother, you're going to be searching a long, long time. You'll find yourself starting and stopping various exercise activities over and over again. As soon as the novelty wears off—which could be within a day or two—and you stop having "fun," you'll be off looking for something else you enjoy. When you fail to make a commitment to do something regularly, you never demonstrate old-fashioned resolve and consistency. You also fail to experience any substantial physical success. Not only are you a "roller-coaster" dieter, you're also a "roller-coaster" exerciser. Get off the roller coaster and get real.

APPENDIX B

Exercises

BODY-WEIGHT EXERCISES

SUMO CHAIR SQUAT

If you had to choose one exercise (you don't), this would be your choice. Sumo Squats exercise your entire lower body, knee to hip, both sides.

HOW ▶

Grab a table chair. Without sitting, straddle the chair with your feet slightly wider than shoulder width and your toes pointed outward. With a slight arch in your lower back and your chest high, lower your body slowly until your butt grazes the chair, then return to the starting position. Do not lock your knees at the top. Grunting is optional.

◀ WHY

What?! Are you kidding me? How about because you enjoy walking. Or maybe being able to ride your bike is of some importance to you. Your legs are your wheels. Take very good care of them.

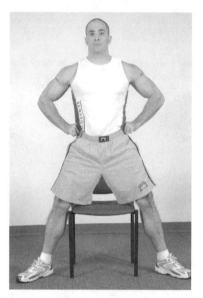 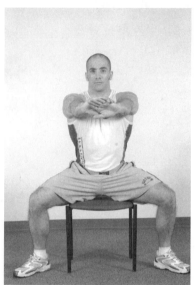

▼ MUSCLES WORKED ▼

Quadriceps—These are the four muscles that comprise the front of your legs.

Gluteus maximus—Your built-in seat cushion. It's a large, powerful muscle.

Hamstrings—The rear or backside of your legs. They attach near the back of your knee and travel all the way up to the pelvis.

THE PROGRAM

The first 30 days—Two sets of twelve repetitions. Rest for twenty seconds between sets.

The next 90 days—Two sets of fifteen repetitions. Rest for twenty seconds between sets.

SUPERMAN

Just breathe naturally. Don't make it complicated.

HOW ▶

Lie facedown on the floor or on a mat (a mat makes it a hell of a lot more comfortable). Form a "T" with your body by extending your arms straight out to the sides. With your head and arms elevated, pull your arms back and slightly up, simultaneously lifting your chest off the mat. Return slowly to the "T" position and repeat.

◀ WHY

All your muscles are important and should be exercised. However, your back is of particular importance. If you want to grow old gracefully and be free of lower back pain, don't neglect your backside.

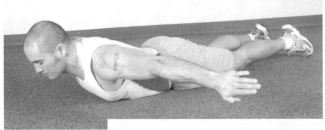

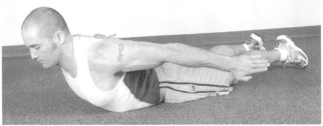

▼ MUSCLES WORKED ▼

Latisimus dorsi—The largest muscles of the back.

Trapezius—The second largest muscle of the back that connects to the base and rear of your skull.

Spinal erectors—Your lower back, big, powerful, and very important.

Gluteus maximus—The ole derriere, your back side, your butt.

Posterior deltoid—The rear of your shoulder.

Triceps—The backs of your arms.

THE PROGRAM

The first 30 days—Two sets of twelve repetitions. Rest for twenty seconds between sets.

The next 90 days—Three sets of fifteen repetitions. Rest for twenty seconds between sets.

PYRAMID PUSHUP

You cannot, nor should you necessarily try, to completely isolate a muscle. The body is designed to operate and function as a collective.

HOW ▶

Get down on your hands and knees. Place your hands on the floor, slightly wider than shoulder width. This exercise is a variation of the old reliable pushup. The primary difference is, instead of having your body completely extended, straight, and on your toes, your feet are going to be substantially closer to your hands. By placing your feet closer to your hands, you must "pike" your torso. Your body should look like an upside down "V" or a pyramid, hence the name.

Holding this position, slowly begin bending your elbows and lowering your forehead to the floor. Attempt to touch it to the floor and then return to the start position. At first, you may have to limit your range of motion by going only a quarter or halfway down. However, each time you exercise, go a little lower and do a few more repetitions. Time is on your side.

◀ WHY

This is a tough exercise, which is one of the reasons I have included it in the program. I prefer this exercise over the old-tried-and-true push-ups because it mimics pushing objects over your head, which clearly reflects our everyday activities.

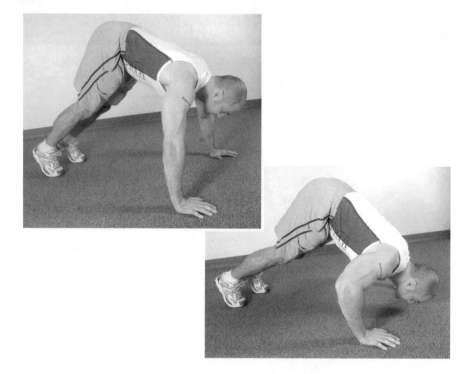

▼ MUSCLES WORKED ▼

Upper pectorals—Your chest, specifically your upper chest.

Anterior deltoid—The front of your shoulders.

Triceps—The rear or backside of your upper arms.

THE PROGRAM

The first 30 days—Two sets of twelve repetitions. Rest for twenty seconds between sets.

The next 90 days—Two sets of fifteen repetitions. Rest for twenty seconds between the sets.

HEAD AND SHOULDER CURL

Train your midsection evenly and proportionately with everything else.

HOW ▶

Lie on your back on the floor or on a mat, with legs together and toes pointed to the ceiling. Place your hands, palms down, under the small of your back. Beginning with your head, slowly roll your torso toward your pelvis, until your elbows also clear the floor. Don't jerk or snap it up. As with all exercises, stay controlled and precise with your movement.

◀ WHY

Lower back pain is at epidemic proportions primarily due to obesity and lack of exercise. The strength of your midsection has a direct relationship to the health of your lower back. Keep your midsection strong for a healthy, happy lower back.

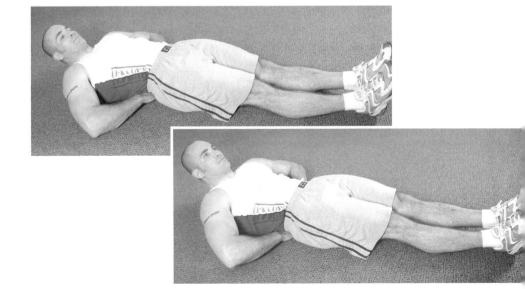

▼ MUSCLES WORKED ▼

Rectus abdominus—Thanks to Britney Spears, Janet Jackson, and Madonna, this muscle (often called the "six pack") has garnered a lot of attention.

External abdominal oblique—Your love handles, or at least, the muscles underneath them.

Serratus anterior—A little bitty muscle that wraps around your upper midsection below your armpits.

THE PROGRAM

The first 30 days—Two sets of twelve repetitions. Rest for twenty seconds between sets.

The next 90 days—Two sets of fifteen repetitions. Rest for twenty seconds between sets.

ARM CIRCLES

Your shoulder joints are the knees of the upper body.
Take good care of them.

HOW ▶

Stand tall with your chest up, your shoulders back, and your knees slightly bent. Extend your arms to the sides so that they are parallel with the floor. Now, imagine you are holding back two walls. Think Hercules. From there, make small tight circles, first backward and then forward.

◀ WHY

Want to change your physique? Change your shoulders. Strong, shapely shoulders are an attractive feature on men and women.

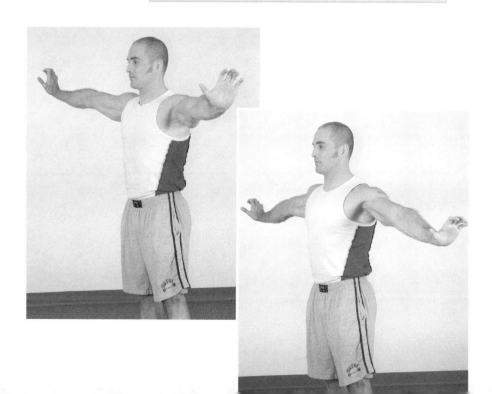

▼ MUSCLES WORKED ▼

Deltoid—The muscle that covers the shoulder joint; it is comprised of three "heads." Your anterior (front), posterior (rear), and medial (side).

Trapezius—Specifically your upper traps; the two muscles of your upper back.

THE PROGRAM

The first 30 days—Not applicable.

The next 90 days—Two sets of fifteen repetitions. Rest twenty seconds between sets.

WEIGHT-TRAINING EXERCISES

FLAT-BENCH DUMBBELL PRESS

Work on lifting your ribcage while performing this exercise.
Vacuum your stomach and keep your chest up.

HOW ▶

Lie back on the bench with your back flat and your feet
flat on the floor. Hold the dumbbells at your sides, with
your elbows at 90-degree angles. Slowly, to a count of
three, press the dumbbells up and together, stopping just
shy of locking your elbows. Slowly return the dumbbells
to the starting position. (Be sure to control the movement—slowly count to three on the way up and down.)

◀ WHY

Because someday you may find yourself pinned
under a car, a candy machine, or your spouse!
If you've been diligent and consistent with this
exercise, you may be able to press your way out.

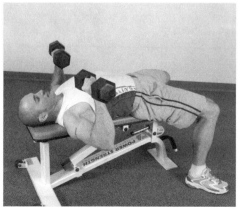
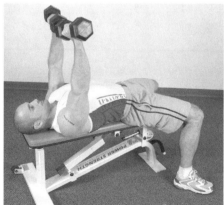

▼ MUSCLES WORKED ▼

Pectorals—Your chest muscles attach at your sternum, stretch across your ribcage, and attach near the armpits.

Anterior and medial deltoid—The flat-bench dumbbell press involves nearly the entire shoulder, including to a limited degree, the rear of your shoulders.

Triceps—Three muscles that comprise the back of your arm.

THE PROGRAM

The first 60 days—Not applicable.

The third 30 days—Two sets of twelve to fifteen repetitions. Rest for twenty to thirty seconds between sets.

The fourth 30 days—Three sets of twelve to fifteen repetitions. Rest for twenty to thirty seconds between sets.

OVERHEAD DUMBBELL PRESS

Stand tall with your abs tight. Use your midsection for support.

HOW ▶

Stand upright, with your feet shoulder width apart. Don't stand with your knees locked. Instead, maintain a slight bend in your knees throughout the exercise. Holding the dumbbells at ear level, slowly press to a full extension above your head. Again, and with all exercises, stop just before your elbows lock. (Be sure to control the movement—slowly count to three on the way up and down.)

◀ WHY

Because the reality is if you don't use them, you'll lose them. It's not just a saying, it's a fact. Muscles simply go away if they're not exercised.

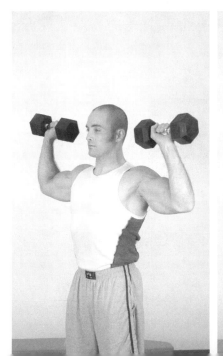 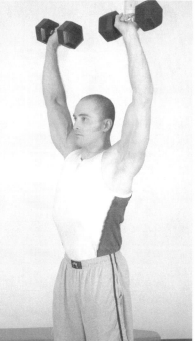

▼ MUSCLES WORKED ▼

Deltoid—Forget about shoulder pads. With this exercise, you make your own.

Upper pectorals—This exercise gets a little help from your upper chest.

Triceps—Sometimes referred to as "horseshoes" because, when nicely developed, this muscle resembles them.

THE PROGRAM

The first 60 days—Not applicable.

The third 30 days—Two sets of twelve to fifteen repetitions. Rest for twenty to thirty seconds between sets.

The fourth 30 days—Three sets of twelve to fifteen repetitions. Rest for twenty to thirty seconds between sets.

TWO-ARM DUMBBELL ROW

**Learn to keep your lower back arched during this exercise.
Lift your chest, arch your lower back, and stick your butt out.**

HOW ▶

Stand with your feet slightly wider than shoulder width.
Bend your knees, lean forward, and sit back with your
butt (without actually sitting!). Your weight should be
evenly centered over your feet. With dumbbells hanging
at arms length, slowly pull them up and toward your
belly button keeping your elbows close to your side.
(Be sure to control the movement—slowly count to
three on the way up and down.)

◀ WHY

Your back is comprised of a lot of muscle. A lot of
important muscle. Your back strength has a direct
relationship to the fitness level of your spine. And in
case you didn't know, your spine is fairly important.

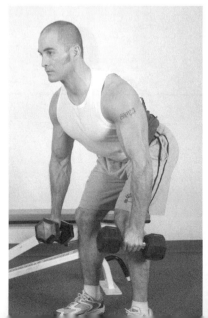
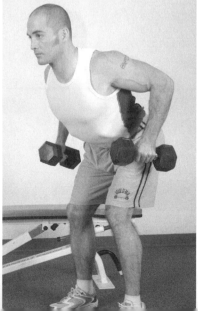

▼ MUSCLES WORKED ▼

Latisimus dorsi—Your "wings."

Trapezoid—Large back muscle that runs from the base of your skull, almost shoulder to shoulder, and down to the middle of your back, attaching on the spine.

Posterior deltoid—The rear muscle that is one of three that comprises your deltoid.

Biceps—Your "GUNS"! Your pythons.

THE PROGRAM

The first 60 days—Not applicable.

The third 30 days—Two sets of twelve to fifteen repetitions. Rest for twenty to thirty seconds between sets.

The fourth 30 days—Three sets of twelve to fifteen repetitions. Rest for twenty to thirty seconds between sets.

BENCH SQUAT

Squats will also work your cardio system. More
than any other exercise, you'll find your breathing and
heart rate increases significantly during squats.

HOW ▶

On the Sumo Chair Squats you used a slightly wider than
shoulder-width stance with toes exaggerated outward.
With Bench Squats, you'll take a shoulder width stance
with toes only slightly and comfortably turned out. Then,
as if sitting on a chair, squat down and slightly back until
your butt grazes the bench. Return to the starting position,
stopping just short of locking your knees. Use your arms as
counterbalance by extending them. (Be sure to control the
movement—slowly count to three on the way up and down.)

◀ WHY

Do you like getting on and off the old
hopper, the thrown, the STOOL with grace?

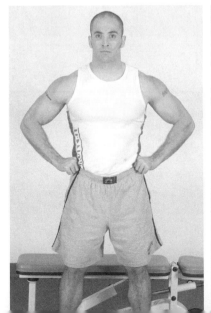
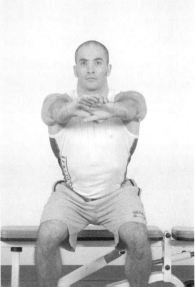

▼ MUSCLES WORKED ▼

Quadriceps—These are the four muscles that comprise the front of your legs.

Gluteus maximus—Your built-in seat cushion. It's a large powerful muscle.

Hamstrings—The rear or backside of your legs. They attach near the rear of your knee, and travel all the way up to the pelvis.

THE PROGRAM

The first 60 days—Not applicable.

The third 30 days—Two sets of twelve to fifteen repetitions. Rest for twenty to thirty seconds between sets.

The fourth 30 days—Three sets of twelve to fifteen repetitions. Rest for twenty to thirty seconds between sets.

BUTT-UP SUPERSETTED WITH REACH-THROUGH CRUNCH

These two exercises are done back to back, first the butt-up then the reach-through crunch, rest and repeat.

HOW ▶

Lying on your back, with your knees bent and feet flat on the floor, raise your pelvis to create a straight line with your body from knees to shoulders. Then return to the starting position. (I like to do butt-ups on a bench, but you could just as easily do them on the floor.)

Now, from the starting position, extend your arms with one hand over the other, spread your knees slightly, and slowly roll up your head and shoulders, reaching through your legs. Return to starting position, and repeat sequence. (Be sure to control the movement—slowly count to three on the way up and down.)

◀ WHY
Butt and abs, baby.
Butt and abs.

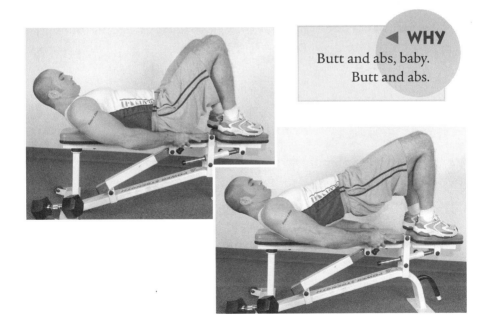

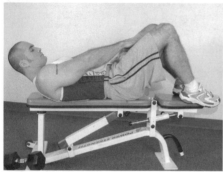
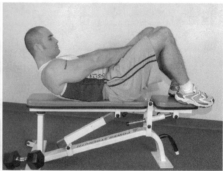

▼ MUSCLES WORKED ▼

Gluteus maximus—Haven't we said enough about this poor muscle already?

Hamstrings—Often neglected but never forgotten. Don't forget to work the backside of your legs.

Rectus abdominus—Your abs.

External abdominal oblique—Your sides.

Serratus anterior—Little bitty muscle that wraps around your upper midsection.

THE PROGRAM

The first 60 days—Not applicable.

The third 30 days—Two sets of twelve to fifteen repetitions. Rest for twenty to thirty seconds between sets.

The fourth 30 days—Three sets of twelve to fifteen repetitions. Rest for twenty to thirty seconds between sets.

APPENDIX C

Workout Schedule

STEP ONE

It is common sense to take a method and try it.
If it fails, admit it frankly and try another.
But above all, try something.

—FRANKLIN D. ROOSEVELT (1882–1945)

DAYS		Sumo Chair Squats (2 x 12)	Pyramid Push-ups (2 x 12)	Supermans (2 x 12)	Head & Shoulder Curls (2 x 12)
EXERCISE PROGRAM • DAYS 1–30					
Mon	SETS				
	REPS				
Thu	SETS				
	REPS				
Mon	SETS				
	REPS				
Thu	SETS				
	REPS				

DAYS		Sumo Chair Squats (2 x 12)	Pyramid Push-ups (2 x 12)	Supermans (2 x 12)	Head & Shoulder Curls (2 x 12)
Mon	SETS				
	REPS				
Thu	SETS				
	REPS				
Mon	SETS				
	REPS				
Thu	SETS				
	REPS				
Mon	SETS				
	REPS				
Thu	SETS				
	REPS				

First do your ten minutes of cardio (stairs, bike, walk, whatever).

Two sets of twelve repetitions is your goal for each exercise. However, in the beginning, you may fall short of twelve repetitions. That's okay. The next workout is another opportunity, and you should strive each time to reach twelve repetitions. In the chart provided, mark how many repetitions you actually do.

Carefully review the exercise photographs to be sure you understand the motions.

Pyramid Push-Ups are probably the hardest of the suggested exercises. In the beginning, you may not be able to touch your forehead to the floor. Each time you perform a push-up, try to get your forehead a little closer to the floor. You'll eventually get stronger and lower. Trust me.

Take twenty to thirty seconds of rest between each set.

It's not absolutely necessary to perform the exercises in the sequence suggested. You could very well perform them in any arrangement. Just do them.

STEP TWO

I was always looking outside myself
for strength and confidence,
but it comes from within.
It is there all the time.

—ANNA FREUD (1895–1982)

	EXERCISE PROGRAM • DAYS 31–60*				
DAYS	Sumo Chair Squats (3 x 15)	Pyramid Push-ups (3 x 15)	Supermans (3 x 15)	Head & Shoulder Curls (3 x 15)	Arm Circles (3 x 15)
Mon SETS					
Mon REPS					
Wed SETS					
Wed REPS					
Fri SETS					
Fri REPS					
Mon SETS					
Mon REPS					
Wed SETS					
Wed REPS					
Fri SETS					
Fri REPS					
Mon SETS					
Mon REPS					
Wed SETS					
Wed REPS					
Fri SETS					
Fri REPS					

DAYS		Sumo Chair Squats (3 x 15)	Pyramid Push-ups (3 x 15)	Supermans (3 x 15)	Head & Shoulder Curls (3 x 15)	Arm Circles (3 x 15)
Mon	SETS					
	REPS					
Wed	SETS					
	REPS					
Fri	SETS					
	REPS					
Mon	SETS					
	REPS					
Wed	SETS					
	REPS					
Fri	SETS					
	REPS					

As with the first thirty days, first do your cardio. But now, do it for a total of fifteen minutes not ten minutes.

Your new goal for each set is fifteen repetitions.

Three-day weekends sometimes interfere with Friday workouts. If you can't work out on Friday, do your workout on Thursday morning. Just don't miss workouts—EVER!

Take twenty to thirty seconds of rest between sets.

Your new exercise is Arm Circles.

STEP THREE

Do not dwell in the past,
do not dream of the future,
concentrate the mind
on the present moment.

—BUDDHA

	EXERCISE PROGRAM • DAYS 61–90				
	Body-weight Exercises				
DAYS	Sumo Chair Squats (3 x 15)	Pyramid Push-ups (3 x 15)	Supermans (3 x 15)	Head & Shoulder Curls (3 x 15)	Arm Circles (3 x 15)
Mon SETS					
Mon REPS					
Wed SETS					
Wed REPS					
Fri SETS					
Fri REPS					
Mon SETS					
Mon REPS					
Wed SETS					
Wed REPS					
Fri SETS					
Fri REPS					
Mon SETS					
Mon REPS					
Wed SETS					
Wed REPS					
Fri SETS					
Fri REPS					

Body-weight Exercises (continued)

DAYS		Sumo Chair Squats (3 x 15)	Pyramid Push-ups (3 x 15)	Supermans (3 x 15)	Head & Shoulder Curls (3 x 15)	Arm Circles (3 x 15)
Mon	SETS					
	REPS					
Wed	SETS					
	REPS					
Fri	SETS					
	REPS					
Mon	SETS					
	REPS					
Wed	SETS					
	REPS					
Fri	SETS					
	REPS					

Weight-lifting Exercises

DAYS		Flat Bench Dumbbell Press (2 x 12–15)	Standing Overhead Dumbbell Press (2 x 12–15)	Two Arm Dumbbell Row (2 x 12–15)	Bench Squats (2 x 12–15)	Butt-ups and Reach-Through Crunches (2 x 12–15)
Mon	SETS					
	REPS					
Wed	SETS					
	REPS					
Fri	SETS					
	REPS					
Mon	SETS					
	REPS					
Wed	SETS					
	REPS					
Fri	SETS					
	REPS					

	Flat Bench Dumbbell Press (2 x 12–15)	Standing Overhead Dumbbell Press (2 x 12–15)	Two Arm Dumbbell Row (2 x 12–15)	Bench Squats (2 x 12–15)	Butt-ups and Reach-Through Crunches (2 x 12–15)
DAYS					

Weight-lifting Exercises (continued)

DAYS		Flat Bench Dumbbell Press (2 x 12–15)	Standing Overhead Dumbbell Press (2 x 12–15)	Two Arm Dumbbell Row (2 x 12–15)	Bench Squats (2 x 12–15)	Butt-ups and Reach-Through Crunches (2 x 12–15)
Mon	SETS					
	REPS					
Wed	SETS					
	REPS					
Fri	SETS					
	REPS					
Mon	SETS					
	REPS					
Wed	SETS					
	REPS					
Fri	SETS					
	REPS					
Mon	SETS					
	REPS					
Wed	SETS					
	REPS					
Fri	SETS					
	REPS					

First do your fifteen minutes of cardio.

Do your body-weight exercises on Wednesdays.

Replace the body-weight exercises you were doing on Fridays with the weight-lifting exercises.

Carefully review the exercise photographs to be sure you understand the motions.

Control the movement. The positive (up) and negative (down) aspects of the exercises should be at the same speed—SLOW! Slowly count to three on the way up and on the way down.

Forget about the amount of weight you're using. Learn to "feel" your muscles.

STEP FOUR

It is courage, courage, courage,
that raises the blood of life to crimson splendor.
Live bravely and present a brave front to adversity.

—HORACE

EXERCISE PROGRAM • DAYS 91–120

Body-weight Exercises

DAYS		Sumo Chair Squats (3 x 15)	Pyramid Push-ups (3 x 15)	Supermans (3 x 15)	Head & Shoulder Curls (3 x 15)	Arm Circles (3 x 15)
Mon	SETS					
	REPS					
Wed	SETS					
	REPS					
Fri	SETS					
	REPS					
Mon	SETS					
	REPS					
Wed	SETS					
	REPS					
Fri	SETS					
	REPS					

Body-weight Exercises (continued)

DAYS		Sumo Chair Squats (3 x 15)	Pyramid Push-ups (3 x 15)	Supermans (3 x 15)	Head & Shoulder Curls (3 x 15)	Arm Circles (3 x 15)
Mon	SETS					
	REPS					
Wed	SETS					
	REPS					
Fri	SETS					
	REPS					
Mon	SETS					
	REPS					
Wed	SETS					
	REPS					
Fri	SETS					
	REPS					
Mon	SETS					
	REPS					
Wed	SETS					
	REPS					
Fri	SETS					
	REPS					

Weight-lifting Exercises

DAYS		Flat Bench Dumbbell Press (2 x 12–15)	Standing Overhead Dumbbell Press (2 x 12–15)	Two Arm Dumbbell Row (2 x 12–15)	Bench Squats (2 x 12–15)	Butt-ups and Reach-Through Crunches (2 x 12–15)
Mon	SETS					
	REPS					
Wed	SETS					
	REPS					
Fri	SETS					
	REPS					

Weight-lifting Exercises (continued)

DAYS		Flat Bench Dumbbell Press (2 x 12–15)	Standing Overhead Dumbbell Press (2 x 12–15)	Two Arm Dumbbell Row (2 x 12–15)	Bench Squats (2 x 12–15)	Butt-ups and Reach-Through Crunches (2 x 12–15)
Mon	SETS					
	REPS					
Wed	SETS					
	REPS					
Fri	SETS					
	REPS					
Mon	SETS					
	REPS					
Wed	SETS					
	REPS					
Fri	SETS					
	REPS					
Mon	SETS					
	REPS					
Wed	SETS					
	REPS					
Fri	SETS					
	REPS					
Mon	SETS					
	REPS					
Wed	SETS					
	REPS					
Fri	SETS					
	REPS					

First do your fifteen minutes of cardio.

Carefully review the exercise photographs to be sure you understand the motions.

Control the movement. The positive (up) and negative (down) aspects of the exercises should be at the same speed—SLOW! Slowly count to three on the way up and on the way down.

Forget about the amount of weight you're using. Learn to "feel" your muscles.

APPENDIX D

Sample Daily Menu and Recipes

SAMPLE DAILY MENU

Breakfast

- 3 egg whites plus one yolk cooked with fat-free and calorie-free cooking spray
- 1 small bowl plain slow-cooking oatmeal
- 1 large glass of water
- 1 cup of coffee (with non-fat or low-fat milk)
- 1 multivitamin/mineral

Mid-Morning Snack

- 1 cup low-carb, low-calorie, low-fat yogurt
- 1 large glass of water

Lunch

- A large green salad with a few strips of grilled chicken
- "Tons" of vegetables and a tablespoon or two of low-calorie dressing
- 1 slice whole-wheat bread
- 1 large glass of water or unsweetened tea

Mid-Afternoon Snack

$\frac{1}{4}$ cup of almonds

1 palm-sized serving of beef jerky

1 large glass of water or unsweetened tea

Supper (as it's known in the heartland)

1 palm-sized serving of chicken, turkey, or fish

2 large servings of green vegetables

Late-Night Snack

2 palm-sized servings steamed Edamame (soybean in the pod).

This is a *sample* menu. You'll have to tailor your eating to your specific tastes and needs. That doesn't mean you should have a Twinkie for breakfast because you need a sugar fix and like the way it tastes! Try different healthy foods to find ones that you like. It really isn't that hard to eat healthy, but it does come with some sacrifice. You have to retrain your taste buds and practice a little patience.

You'd probably like me to script out about ten or more daily meal plans, but I just won't do it. Why not? Because I don't think you'll learn from it, and if you don't learn, your success—if you experience any—will be short and fleeting. You'll only learn by doing for yourself. So go ahead and make up some sample menus on your own.

Cook with fat-free cooking sprays.

Use fat-free and low-calorie dressings and sauces.

Splenda is a wonderful sweetener. Use it, and throw away the sugar.

Don't count calories.

Make better food choices.

Cook more often.

Eat LOTS of vegetables. They're virtually calorie-free and are loaded with nutrients!

**Forget the word *diet*. It's NOT a DIET! It's a *lifestyle*!
Diet is a short-term program . . . lifestyle is forever!**

ORIGINAL GOYA RECIPES

Anytime Omelet

Nonstick cooking spray

3–6 egg whites* or
egg substitute

Garlic powder to taste

Italian seasoning to taste

2 tsp grated Parmesan cheese

2–3 slices honey-smoked
turkey breast

Unlimited veggies of choice

2 tablespoons pasta sauce (optional)

*Add one yolk per three egg whites, if desired

Set burner on medium heat. Spray medium-sized pan with nonstick cooking spray. Pour in eggs or egg substitute and allow egg to spread in pan. Setting aside the sauce, place all other ingredients evenly over the eggs. When the eggs are opaque, flip over "pancake-style" and cook until slightly browned. Remove from heat. Sprinkle sauce over one side of the omelet and fold in half.

Banana Protein Pancakes

1/4 cup whole-wheat pancake mix

2 scoops vanilla whey-protein
powder

6 egg whites*

1 very ripe banana

1/3 cup low-fat cottage cheese

1 tbsp Splenda

1 tsp vanilla

Nonstick cooking spray,
butter-flavored

1/4 cup crushed or
chopped walnuts (optional)

*Add one yolk per three egg whites, if desired

In a blender, combine all ingredients except walnuts. Blend until smooth. Preheat a nonstick griddle over medium heat. Coat with non-fat butter-flavored cooking spray. Pour portions of batter onto griddle. When topside becomes bubbly, flip pancakes and cook until done. Top with walnuts, if desired.

Turkey Parmesan

4–5 turkey breast or cutlets

2 egg whites

1 cup Italian-flavored bread crumbs or crushed croutons

2 tsp olive oil or nonstick cooking spray

1 cup chunky pasta sauce

2–3 tsp grated Parmesan cheese

1/8–1/4 cup Italian-style 6-Cheese Blend or similar product

Preheat oven to 350 degrees. Dip meat in egg whites and coat with bread crumbs or croutons. Preheat a nonstick griddle over medium heat. Coat with nonstick cooking spray or olive oil. Pan sear turkey pieces until browned on both sides. Remove from pan and place in baking dish. Cover seared turkey pieces with sauce and cheese. Bake for about 20 minutes.

Turkey/Chicken Burgers

1/2 lbs ground turkey or chicken breast

2 tbsp pasta sauce

1–2 tsp parsley

1–2 tsp onion flakes

1–2 cloves fresh garlic, crushed

2 egg whites

1/2 cup crushed croutons or Italian-style bread crumbs

Setting aside croutons or bread crumbs, mix all ingredients together in a large bowl. Roll individual balls and flatten into patties. Gently press each side of the patties into croutons or bread crumbs. Preheat pan over medium heat. Spray with nonstick cooking spray. Pan sear patties until brown on all sides and cooked through.

Chicken Chili

1 tsp chopped fresh garlic

1 tbsp olive oil

2 12.5-ounce cans of chicken breast

1 14-ounce can fat-free chicken broth

1 14.5-ounce can chopped tomatoes with jalapeño or green chilies

1/2 8-ounce can crisp corn, drained

1 8-ounce can chili beans or black beans, drained

1 8-ounce can white or other bean

1 tsp chili powder

1 tbsp chopped dried onion or chopped fresh onion to taste

Over medium heat, sauté the garlic in olive oil until brown. Begin adding canned ingredients one at a time. Add chili powder and onion. Mix gently. Cook over low to medium heat for about 25 minutes until simmering.

Asian Chicken Salad

1/2 bag broccoli slaw (about 8–10 ounces)

1/2 bag coleslaw (about 8–10 ounces)

1/4 cup finely chopped green onion

1/4 cup chopped red bell pepper

1/4 cup sliced almonds

2 chopped grilled chicken breasts

Basic Dressing

1 tbsp peanut butter

2 tbsp sesame oil

1/2 cup rice wine vinegar

2 tbsp Splenda

Splash of light (low-salt) soy

1/4 cup water

Mix together all salad fixings in a large bowl. To make the dressing, dissolve peanut butter in sesame oil. Add the remaining dressing ingredients and stir well. Drizzle dressing over the salad.

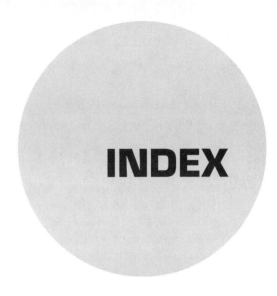

INDEX

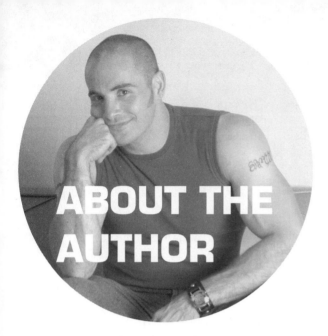

ABOUT THE AUTHOR

Marty Tuley is an author, personal trainer, competitive natural body-builder, and power lifter. He owned and operated a commercial health club for more than ten years. Whether he's training a professional athlete, a homemaker, or a nine-to-fiver, he touts the same exercise message: *It's not about the magic pill or the routine. It's all about dedication, consistency, and plain ole HARD work. Get used to it*!

Marty lives in Lawrence, Kansas, with his wife, Lovena, where they own and operate an exclusive, one-on-one personal-training studio. When they're not at the studio, they're busy spending time with their adopted dogs, Neesha, Blitz, and Bud.

Visit www.getoffyourass.biz

A portion of the proceeds from the sale of this book will be donated to PE4Life to support its mission: inspiring active, healthy living by advancing the development of quality, daily physical education programs for all children. For more information, go to **www.pe4life.com**